DISCARD

Early Praise for
THE DYING TIME

"Written by a consummate nurse and a humane attorney, *The Dying Time* addresses the multitude of everyday questions, concerns, and fears that arise in the process of dying. Preparing for death is a final step in living a healthy life. Furman and McNabb explain the complexity of dying in a simple yet personal voice."

VIRGINIA TROTTER BETTS, M.S.N., J.D., R.N.,
immediate past president, American Nurses Association

"An enormously useful book for caregivers, hospice workers, and anyone who wants to understand the stages of the dying process. This is the clearest and most straightforward text I have read on the subject."

JOAN HALIFAX, PH.D., founder of The Project of Being with Dying

"A manual of immediately practical assistance for humankind's most significant—and often most frightening—moment, death. Besides an enthusiastic response from all who ~~~~~~~~ ~dle their own and others' deaths ~~~~~~~~~~~~~~~~~~~ ~es to be part of the core curricu~~~~~~~~~~~~~~~~~~~ ~d ministry. Already singular in it~~~~~~~~~~~~~~~ *~he Dying Time* will become a class~~~~~~~

GEORGE FOWLER, author of *Dance of a Fallen Monk*

D1042689

The
DYING
TIME

The
DYING
TIME

Practical Wisdom
for the Dying
and Their Caregivers

JOAN FURMAN, M.S.N., R.N.

AND DAVID MCNABB

BELL TOWER
New York

This book is not intended as a substitute for the medical advice of physicians. Any application of the recommendations set forth in this book is at the reader's discretion and sole risk. The reader should regularly consult a doctor in matters relating to health and particularly with respect to symptoms that may require diagnosis or medical attention. All names and identifying information have been changed to protect confidentiality of patients.

Grateful acknowledgment is made to the Institute of Noetic Sciences for the use of the poem "The Last Resort" from *Life's Finishing School* by Helen Green Ansley. Copyright © 1990 by the Institute of Noetic Sciences. Also to Prelude Press for two poems by Peter McWilliams from *How to Survive the Loss of a Love* by Melba Colgrove, Ph.D., Harold H. Bloomfield, M.D., and Peter McWilliams.

Published by Bell Tower, an imprint of Harmony Books, a division of Crown Publishers, Inc., 201 East 50th Street, New York, New York 10022.
Member of the Crown Publishing Group.
Random House, Inc. New York, Toronto, London, Sydney, Auckland
http://www.randomhouse.com/
Bell Tower and colophon are trademarks of Crown Publishers, Inc.

Printed in the United States of America

DESIGN BY DEBORAH KERNER

Library of Congress Cataloging-in-Publication Data is available upon request.

ISBN 0-609-80003-5
10 9 8 7 6 5 4 3 2 1
First Edition

To Michael, whose death changed my life;
to Erin, Sarah, and Dan,
    whose lives stopped my death;
to Lazaris, whose love healed my soul.

                                        Joan

To Daniel J. Goodman,
lover, lawyer, poet, and friend.

And to the others now gone—
Lynn, Fred, Rell, Dick, Evan, David, Grey,
Bill, Denny, Bob, Corey, Arthur, Tom, Greg,
Dorothy, Donald, Joe, Rob, David, Bobby,
Leslie, Glenn, Cardinal, Michael, Chris,
Allen, DeDe, Ed, Michael, Randy, Jan,
Paul, Rusty, Breton—
    who taught me how to live.

May their memories be for a blessing.

                                        David

Contents

Contents

Acknowledgments

Our heartfelt thanks to the patients and friends who have died and have been our greatest teachers.

We would like to express our gratitude to friends and colleagues who gave us the help we needed in writing this book: Nancy Telford, Vicki Slater, Ralph Cadenhead, David Cellon, and Jim Furman. And to the wizards of technology who enabled us to coauthor a book from opposite sides of the country.

We would also like to thank Toinette Lippe, our tireless and patient editor, as well as Lowenstein-Morel Associates, and Eileen Cope, our literary agents, for taking a chance with us. A special thanks to George Fowler, author and monk-at-large, who said, "Maybe I can help." And to Kellogg Fellow Ray Gatchalian, who said, "You need to write this book." Thanks to Drs. Richard Rose, Jeffry King, Ken Lichtenstein and nurse Kay Williams for their wisdom and care of the dying.

Finally we would like to acknowledge Dr. Elisabeth Kübler-Ross, who paved the road for all of us to be free to learn about healing in the dying time and to become midwives of the exit.

Preface

My life's journey, my soul's journey, has always been about healing. The word "healing" comes from the Anglo-Saxon *haelen,*
meaning "to make whole." For me, healing and dying are totally
compatible concepts. To live and die consciously is to walk the
healing path toward wholeness and to live through and accept
dying as a part of life.

I always knew I would be a nurse, then later a nurse practitioner, but it wasn't clear to me that I would become a "spiritual
midwife." However, as a seventeen-year-old freshman nursing
student, I attended my first of over one thousand deaths and
soon thereafter my first of about two thousand births. During
those early years, I lost countless friends in Vietnam, including
a loved one, and by age twenty-three had survived my own near-
death experience. I began to realize that I wanted to make death
less frightening, mysterious, and out of control and more peaceful, loving, and safe for everyone in my care.

As a nurse practitioner, I still work with the dying. I have been fortunate to live my destiny and my purpose in healing the sick and dying, not by curing, but by caring. My hope is that some of the experiences that I describe in this book will help you find your own way of living through the dying time.

Dying and death, just like birthing and birth, are events of such beauty and awesome magnitude that I still cry at every one. The presence of Spirit in the room is palpable with the same intensity at birth or death. Each time I "listen" to the unseen, I sense great celebration in the room. The dying person often seems to be participating in that celebration, even though his body seems still in labor. I try to attend the death of every one of my clients. Like well-coached birthing, well-coached dying is a transcendent experience. The dying time can truly be a time of light and learning for all of us, although for most people it is a time of great fear.

In 1987, in one of those synchronicities that reminds us that there are no accidents, and after a life crisis that set me on a path of growth, I was asked to coordinate the Tennessee AIDS Advisory Committee, where I met David. David and I realized that since all of us have to die, most people would like it to be a positive experience. Hardly anyone knows how to do that, and we wanted to develop a method that helps people through this monumental life phase we call the dying time.

We hope that the experiences of patients (with names and identifying information changed) and friends that we share in this book, as well as the method we have devised, will be meaningful to you. Naturally we bring to this process our personal biases, some of which even David and I struggled to agree upon. In all of this, it is our hope that *The Dying Time* will be valuable in your healing. We wish you peace.

JOAN FURMAN

I grew up in a small town in central Indiana, with a closeness in the community that rarely exists today. In the nurturing environment of an extended family I first learned the qualities of care and service that would stand me in good stead when I became a caregiver. I determined early in life to become a lawyer, and once I had graduated and met my life partner I settled into a nice, middle-class life of law and politics. At that time, the notion that I would end up caring for the dying never entered my head.

In 1981 the first cases of AIDS were reported, though it was not yet known by that name. By 1987 the tidal wave of the epidemic had reached Tennessee, and my friends began to die. Later that year I saw a story on the evening news about the state AIDS Advisory Committee, just set up in Tennessee's health department. The chair of the committee said that she had been unable to get any HIV-positive people to serve on the committee. I called and volunteered my services, and three days later the governor appointed me to the committee.

Life brings many unexpected turns and twists; that is how we learn. Along with my service on the committee, which issued its report in 1988, I began caring for people who were in the hospital and desperately ill. Since then I have taken care of dozens of friends in their dying time and learned caregiving skills from doctors and nurses who are the finest examples of humanity I have known. I have come to realize that dying and living are inseparably intertwined; in a very real way, we begin to die the moment we are born. Since dying is inevitable, we should take care that it is, as far as possible, an experience marked by peace and growth for all concerned.

As Joan and I share our insights from our experiences with the dying, we hope that you gain a better understanding of what is happening to you and how you can deal with all the issues you must face. Serenity, and even joy, may be found at the end of life, and that is what we wish for you.

David McNabb

The
DYING
TIME

✂ *Introduction*

My name is Death:
The last, best friend am I.
ROBERT SOUTHEY

This book offers our vision of the dying time as the last dance of life, one that every single person now living or who will ever live will have to perform. Some people perform this dance with grace and beauty, while for others it is marred by physical and emotional pain. It is our goal to help the dying and their caregivers understand what is happening to them and to assist them in the emotional, physical, and spiritual struggles that occur as the drama is played out.

A word about pronouns. English has few options in pronouns. The use of "he" is irritating for many people, as are the construct of "s/he" and the use of "he or she." To address this, certain chapters use exclusively masculine pronouns, while others are exclusively feminine. This has its drawbacks, but there is really no satisfactory solution to this problem. English also has no word for the feminine aspect of God. We have therefore sometimes used "God or Goddess" to express both the masculine and feminine qualities of the deity.

Sages and philosophers have always counseled that we should live each day as if it were our last, though few have followed this advice. Most people do not want to confront or think about death until they have to. That has resulted, in American culture, in a haphazard approach to the dying process, as if, since everyone has to do it, we all know how to manage it. When you are confronting your own death or that of a loved one, the details of management can be overwhelming.

How do you identify the dying time, and how do you plan for it? Broadly speaking, the dying time begins when someone's physical condition has declined to the point where his continued physical existence is imminently threatened or when he accepts the idea that the condition he has been diagnosed with will soon end his life. The old expression "putting your affairs in order" can be useful, but it usually includes only things like disposing of your property and writing a will. Although we will cover some of those issues in this book, we have broadened the concept to include personal care for you and your caregiver, arranging the details of your dying, recovering your own innate spirituality, repairing your family and other relationships, making funeral arrangements, and grieving.

At the beginning of each chapter, there is advice addressed directly to the person who is dying and to the caregiver. The issues that each faces in the cycle of dying are different but intimately related. When one leaves, another is left. The pain of both is real. Some of the chapters will primarily address one person or the other, but both can benefit from the insights and suggestions.

When a person approaches death, when he has to confront the fact that time is not only limited but measurably so, he has to think about whether there is any continued existence, and if so, what it might be like. Our whole lives are bound up in physical existence. What does it even mean to speak of life on some other plane, in some other dimension? How would we think, how would we feel and experience, without a brain, organs, and the senses?

Those questions cannot be answered finally, with or without a leap of faith. We can assure one another that we know what happens when we die, but this is not the same thing as the knowledge that two plus two equals four. We each have a belief system that corresponds to and grows out of what happens to us. It is the similarity of our lives that allows us to talk to one another about our spiritual experiences. Each of us is in his own place, being created out of, and creating, innumerable and sometimes uncontrollable individual events. We also have our absolute and radical individuality, and it is the combination of the two that makes us human. One such life-changing event reported by many is the "near-death experience," a time when the body is technically in a state of death for a short period of time. Near-death experiences are reported as similar in many respects and often serve as a catalyst in the development of identity and personal spirituality.

Joan: When I was a very young intensive care nurse, recently out of undergraduate school, I had what I later understood to be a near-death experience. I had had a severe case of laryngitis that was causing swelling in my throat. After accidental exposure to a lethal gas, my already irritated throat swelled and my voicebox closed. I had what is known as a laryn-gospasm. Fortunately I was in bed in a hospital when this occurred. I remember the minutes before losing consciousness as the most terrifying moments of my life. Air hunger—gasping for breath—is the most primal of urges, so powerful that I was unaware of anything else going on around me.

The next thing I remember was watching my own resuscitation from the corner of the ceiling. The scene is as vivid today as it was twenty-seven years ago. My limp, unconscious body was on a hospital bed facing me, with two doctors and a nurse on my right side, starting an IV in my right arm at the elbow. I was viewing them from the backs and tops of their heads. I don't remember seeing their faces. On the left side of my body were a doctor and a nurse and the "crash cart." The doctor was prepping my neck for a tracheotomy, and the nurse was drawing up medication into the syringe. I could hear only muffled sounds and felt surprised, because resuscitation efforts are usually very noisy. I heard voices and listened dispassionately to their assessment of the mess everyone thought I was in. I did notice that the doctor who was prepping my neck contaminated his instruments. I thought, Oh, look. He broke sterile technique. Oh, well.

I felt so at peace, so surrounded with love and safety, that I had no desire to return to my body. In fact, I had a detached curiosity about it all. I liked it there at the corner of the ceiling. I did not see relatives who had died before, nor did I see a tunnel of bright light, both frequently reported phenomena of near-death experiences. I wonder now if I would have had those experiences if the resuscitation had not worked so quickly, but I suddenly felt the pain of the resuscitation and knew I was back in my body. I don't know how long that took, and I don't know how I got down from the ceiling. All I knew was that I was miserable in my body and once again terrified and desperate for air. I remember thinking, Why did *this* have to happen?!

I learned some important lessons that day about life and death that helped me deal with the death of a loved one and even today shapes my professional career. I understood with all of my being, not just intellectually, that I am more than my body. My body was a vehicle, and I had literally left. Being out of it produced less sentiment than trading in an old car. I learned that my ability to observe, think, evaluate, and make decisions was not dependent on being in my body. I knew about sterile technique, observed it being broken, evaluated that it wasn't important, and made a decision not to act. I felt love, peace, happiness, contentment, and curiosity, so my ability to feel was still intact. It was as though I knew that what was real was who and where I was, not what was going on in the room below me.

Being trained in the sciences, I wrote off my experience as hypoxic hallucination. I didn't share what had happened even with people I trusted because I didn't believe it myself. Only after similar experiences began to be reported in the professional literature did I believe it myself. Now I can't imagine not believing it. I know that life continues after the death of the body. I trust what happened. It was big, bigger than any other experience I ever had. It changed my life.

ෆ ෆ ෆ ෆ ෆ ෆ ෆ ෆ ෆ ෆ ෆ ෆ ෆ ෆ ෆ ෆ ෆ ෆ ෆ

From all our observations, we believe that death is only a transition, a journey from one state of being to another. Just as the caterpillar must die to become a butterfly, so human beings must go through this stage of metamorphosis. It is different for each of us, but this we know: Though we are different, we are not alone.

In the old days, visiting hours in hospitals were approximately from 7:00 to 7:15 P.M., and caregivers were expected to leave as soon as visiting hours were over. That, thankfully, has become a thing of the past. Good care practices now emphasize the role of family and friends in caring for the sick person, and when someone moves on to the drama of dying, the professional staff is now trained to support the individual caregivers instead of shutting them out. Also, the rise of the hospice movement, with its emphasis on pain relief and the dignity of dying, has radically reshaped our notions of what the physical side of the dying time will be like.

There is still, unfortunately, a reluctance to talk about the actual process of dying. Even our funerals, as a rule, try to hide the reality that someone has died. The casket is covered with flowers. We never actually see the grave filled in or the cremation being performed, and people avoid mentioning that a death has occurred, lest someone become emotionally upset. More traditional societies have a different and altogether healthier approach, treating dying as part of living. In America, with our emphasis on youth, vitality, and physical beauty, we see death as the enemy; the end of physical existence as being the end of everything of value. Our bias as a culture for competition and winning makes death a symbol of failure.

Death is not just an end, but a new beginning. Wherever we came from, and wherever we are going, is not in our hands. We may delay, but we can never truly cheat death. It comes for everyone. In the process of dying, the opportunity presents itself to make a final testament to a life well lived, to resolve any bitterness that may have grown between yourself and others, and to leave a recognition with the living that your human experience had dignity and value. In order to do this, we suggest that you take responsibility for the arrangements of your dying in the same way and to the same degree that you have taken responsibility for your living arrangements. You can decide where the event will take place, of course taking into account your physical condition and that of your caregiver. You can decide what course your medical treatment should take. You can decide who will be with you, what your environment will be like, what music you will hear, what you will look upon. You cannot change the fact of death, but you can have a great deal of control over the how, when, and where of it. That is your responsibility, to yourself and to your loved ones. If you are not physically capable of that degree of effort, then one or all of your loved ones can be brought into the process. This is your last opportunity to reveal your mind and spirit, to allow those you love to see you as you truly are.

When people are ill, they tend to become passive, and this increases with the severity of the illness. For those suffering from long-term disease, the process of withdrawal from the world of the living can extend over many months. This may inhibit you or your caregivers in making arrangements for your actual death, causing you to avoid conversations with loved ones that you believe might cause them pain. This pain is unavoidable, but it is honest and clean and part of the process. The dying person has to summon the courage and grace to leave this life, and his loved ones have to go on living.

As death approaches, you will find that you do withdraw from the living world. This drama we call death is like a play. You are both the playwright and the director. You decide what staging will be used, who will play what roles, who will speak and who will remain silent. If your loved ones, who will be providing your care, know about your decisions in advance, then you can rest easy knowing that your wishes will be followed. You can then concentrate on living the remaining time that you have. Just as when you prepare for a journey, you must pack, make arrangements for the dog, and mentally check the thousand details that present themselves, so too when you die you must prepare yourself. But also just as you would not set out on a journey by trusting to fate and chance to get where you wanted to go, so in dying you should not be just a passive spectator or someone else will have to take charge. No one else can know your mind unless you express it. That can be a frightening process, because in revealing yourself, you become vulnerable. It is your right to make as many decisions as possible, and it is also your duty. Just as you have many issues to resolve in confronting death, so do your loved ones.

Introducing the dying time would not be complete without discussing the concept of "being" for the caregiver. The "doing" focus is the part of us that is what we call masculine energy. Sometimes this "doing" energy is spent physically performing all the tasks that provide physical comfort to the one who is ill. The feminine part, the "being" focus, is often left out or is unnoticed. (By masculine and feminine, we are not referring to male or female. All humans have both kinds of abilities or energy, and they are equally important.) Discussion of this feminine aspect is usually met with the question "But how do you do 'being'?"

"Being" is the love, the compassion, the genuine concern, the "being with" another. It is giving that person your full attention, the greatest gift you can give, holding nothing back for yourself. It is actually a very active energy, but is seldom seen, or is viewed as less important. It is the creation of the safety for your loved one to explore his emotional and spiritual healing. It is creating the environment in which healing and wholeness can occur, regardless of what forms they take. It is perceiving the needs and conceiving the plans for action to alleviate discomfort. It is empowering for your loved one to stay in charge of his living and dying, thus ensuring his dignity. It is allowing the transition and being with him in awe and in wonder and also in pain and loss. Sometimes it looks as though nothing at all is happening, and that may be the most important time. It reminds us of the old adage "Don't just do something, stand there." There are times when there seems to be nothing to do or nothing that one can do because the situation seems impossible. At those times we need to accept our helplessness and not fight against it. Our ability to do this will provide a foundation and background for acceptance on the part of the dying person. There may indeed *be* nothing to do, except be there to see or, as some say, to bear witness to the life of another. The last moments of life are precious, and being with the dying moment by moment is perhaps the most important thing.

ⓘⓘⓘ ⓘⓘⓘ ⓘⓘⓘ ⓘⓘⓘ ⓘⓘⓘ ⓘⓘⓘ ⓘⓘⓘ ⓘⓘⓘ ⓘⓘⓘ ⓘⓘⓘ ⓘⓘⓘ ⓘⓘⓘ ⓘⓘⓘ ⓘⓘⓘ ⓘⓘⓘ ⓘⓘⓘ ⓘⓘⓘ ⓘⓘⓘ

Joan: Jim and Susan were an elderly couple who had been married for fifty-three years when she was diagnosed with very advanced leukemia. Their relationship was strong, and they were very close and comfortable with each other. When Susan became ill, Jim went into a frenzy of studying every book, every source he and I could find about cancer, its traditional as well as complementary therapies. He orchestrated her diet, her access to negative people and written materials, her food supplements, and her many choices of alternative treatments. He drove her, took care of her, and was her champion. In fact, Susan and I had to work on setting limits on his making decisions for her, which he agreed to with a sheepish grin! No obstacle was too great for him, and he cared for Susan beautifully all through her treatment and dying process. His strength was his ability to use that masculine energy to get the job done.

However, in the last few days of Susan's life, when there seemed to be nothing left for him to *do* (to prevent her death, his "job"), he couldn't find a role for himself. He had been so focused on trying to save her life that when it became apparent that that was no longer possible, he was unaware that he had anything left to contribute. His "doing" job was over; he felt useless. Sadly, Jim left an hour before Susan's death finally occurred. He forgot to call me to her deathbed, even though she had requested that I be present and had asked him to be sure I was notified. He simply saw the failure of his work, the loss of the goal that he had had, and the uselessness of any further activity.

This is a perfect example of a person with a beautiful masculine energy and a complete unawareness of his feminine side. His behavior was not an indication of his lack of love; that was strong. He simply believed he had no further role. Being with her quietly during the last breath and heartbeat of her life might have comforted her even though she was no longer conscious, and it would certainly have provided him with comfort later in his bereavement. This was an opportunity lost.

ﻩﻩﻩ ﻩﻩﻩ ﻩﻩﻩ ﻩﻩﻩ ﻩﻩﻩ ﻩﻩﻩ ﻩﻩﻩ ﻩﻩﻩ ﻩﻩﻩ ﻩﻩﻩ ﻩﻩﻩ ﻩﻩﻩ ﻩﻩﻩ ﻩﻩﻩ ﻩﻩﻩ ﻩﻩﻩ ﻩﻩﻩ ﻩﻩﻩ ﻩﻩﻩ

You are about to set out on the ultimate journey. With regrets and sorrow, yes, but also with a sense of anticipation. If we can help you on this journey in any small way, it will be our pleasure and our joy to have brought you this book.

1 ✂ *Choices*

My comfort is my only concern.
DANIEL J. GOODMAN, 1949–1994

To the One Facing Death   ✂

When most people contemplate the circumstances of their own death, what becomes apparent is that they do not necessarily fear death itself, but the loss of control and dignity that is proper to living beings. Studies have shown that if you ask people whether they want to die in a hospital or on a ventilator, almost everyone says, "No." In this chapter we will look at some of the choices you will be faced with and where those choices are likely to lead. One key to achieving a certain level of serenity can be to talk about your approaching death, either with your family or other people whom you trust, and to take some control of the dying time.

To the Caregiver ≈

The drama of dying is a play in which there are many actors, all of whom are important, but there is only one director, and that is the one who is facing death. He is the one who should be writing the script, if he is able to do so. You can assist him in this process by being open about your feelings, by listening to him, and by making every effort to arrange things as he wishes, from funeral preparations to the more wrenching decisions concerning medical treatment and nursing care. If everyone in the drama reads from the same script, much of the chaos that can occur will be avoided and the death will more likely have meaning and dignity. While everyone involved in your loved one's care will be under a lot of stress, and especially those whom he loves, it remains a fact that he must at all times be consulted about any arrangements for his care. Now, it is possible that he may become very passive about such issues and won't want to be involved in the decision-making process; that in itself can be a decision. Be aware, however, that barring a coma, he may at seemingly odd times (and over minor issues) seek to assert some control. Try to be attentive at those times and respectful, as much as possible, of his wishes. This can be difficult, since he may express himself with anger or apparent spitefulness. Through the anger, you can reach a level of communication that otherwise might not occur because of your loved one's passivity.

In the event that your loved one is unable or unwilling to direct the process, that duty will of necessity devolve upon the caregivers, who should be prepared with a durable power of attorney to give them the legal right to make such decisions relating to the health care of the dying person. That issue and other legal questions are discussed in this chapter, along with many other decisions that will need to be made.

Home, Hospital, or Hospice ✂

Many factors are involved in deciding where the dying should occur. First and foremost will be the physical condition of your loved one. It may not be possible for him to be at home because of the volume of medication he is receiving, his condition, or the lack of local hospice or home health agencies. Also, the capabilities of the caregivers at home can be crucial in this decision. The caregivers may not have the physical stamina necessary to provide the kind of care at home that will be needed. Home health or hospice nurses cannot be present all the time, and if your loved one's physical needs will be too demanding for you, then a setting other than the home may be more appropriate. However, there are important reasons for him to remain in the home, if that is possible.

First, he will be less agitated and emotionally more serene if he is in familiar surroundings. Being in a comforting and normal environment can help him remain mentally focused. It is more convenient for the caregivers, since they know where everything is, children do not have to be arranged for, pets can be let out, and the caregivers can sleep in their own beds. The kitchen is immediately available and stocked with food that everyone likes.

On the other hand, a hospital or other health care facility, including a residential hospice, if available, has many advantages, including an unlimited supply of clean bed linens, immediate access to pain and stress relievers, and a trained staff to assist you. Your loved one may be receiving intravenous medication, in considerable pain, or incontinent. If he is uncomfortable at home, or if you are unable to care for him effectively, then you need to consider the alternatives. It is not a defeat to recognize where the dying person will be most comfortable. For many of the dying, being sent to the hospital or out of the home is a sure sign that death is imminent, when that is not necessarily the case.

This decision about the location for a dying time must be discussed with the person who is dying, if that is possible. If he is still in denial about his condition, talk about the death scene may be most unwelcome, but there are several methods that may help your loved one to open up about his fears and concerns. A dying person will not talk about the issues surrounding death until he is ready to do so. He may want to discuss his death but may be reluctant to do so, for fear of upsetting those around him. During a conversation about how his condition is worsening, you could try asking any of these questions: (1) "It seems as though things aren't going so well for you right now. What do you think is going on?" (2) "Do you think your body is beginning to let go?" (3) "Where do you think you would like to be if your health starts to get worse?" (4) "If you start having more problems with your (pain, breathing, self-care, etc.), would you like to be at home or in a hospital?" In this way, your loved one's need for acknowledging hope for his condition is expressed without stripping away his control and dignity.

A more indirect approach may sometimes be useful. Perhaps you both know someone who has died, maybe on a respirator. You could bring up the subject, and your loved one may quite directly say, "I sure don't want anything like that to happen to me!" A general discussion about whether you would like to be taken care of in the home if the situations were reversed might allow him to make his wishes known, again without abandoning his sense of safety. In this way he avoids having to confront the fact that his own death is approaching.

Even so, usually at some time in the process of dying, your loved one will reach the point that he wants and needs to talk about his death. He may still not wish to discuss the details, so you will have to make many decisions without his guidance. While this is regrettable, it is not unusual for this to happen. While the methods just discussed may provide an opening to the dying person to discuss his death, it is by no means certain that he will choose to do so. The most that you can do is to remain open to the discussion of his dying and to let him know you are available to talk when and if he wishes to. The moment may come immediately prior to his death or days, weeks, or even months beforehand.

If your loved one expresses a strong desire to remain at home during the dying time, then every effort should be made to comply with those wishes. If there are not sufficient caregivers in the home, find out from the hospital social workers or the doctor or nurses where more professional help can be obtained. Many insurance companies, in an effort to reduce costs, can be quite cooperative in paying for additional nursing in the home if it keeps the dying person out of the hospital. Round-the-clock nursing in the home is cheaper than being in the hospital.

As a caregiver, be aware that help is usually available, not only professionally, but also personally. Your friends and associates, and those of your loved one, may be unaware that you need help. Many people feel awkward about being around the dying. Even though they are willing to help, they don't know what to do or what you need to have done. It is likely that they will say something like "If I can do anything, let me know." You may find that unhelpful, since you don't really know by that statement what they are truly willing to do and if you would be imposing on their generosity. They may be willing to do some shopping for you but may not want to assume responsibility for the care of your loved one for a period of time so that you can leave. We have found that the best approach is for you to be up front about what you need and let your friends decide for themselves what they can do to help you. If you need something from the store, then by all means say so when someone asks what he can do. If you need some time out of the house, perhaps he would be willing to come to the house for a couple of hours so that you can do that.

If it is not possible for the dying person to stay at home, then explain to him the factors that are driving the decision; he may himself be able to suggest ways to get around the difficulties. The most important thing to do is listen. You may discover his feelings on a whole range of subjects, and he may in the end convince himself that the hospital or one of the other facilities is the appropriate place to be. Try to be sensitive to what he is telling you and avoid announcing the decision as if there are no alternatives, which will make it seem as though he is losing control of his life. The key is consultation and listening and investigating all of the available options for help so that the facts of the situation will be clear to you both.

A word about hospice care. More and more communities have hospice available, either residential or in the home. The staff of these facilities are trained specifically to help the dying make their transition in physical comfort and emotional and spiritual serenity. They are experts in pain management and are aware that good nursing care continues until and even beyond death. Nursing is a profession of caring, and caring is as relevant after therapeutic treatment has been stopped as before, or even more so.

Good nursing is vital for pain management, supervision of physical care, provision of emotional support for the dying one and his caregivers, and preparation of the dying and his family and loved ones for the transition of death. Hospice organizations also frequently have aides available who are trained in the physical care of the dying, and they can come to your home to look after your loved one for a period of hours so that you can take a break.

Curing or Healing

Medical care of people with life-threatening illness can have two goals: curing and recovery, or comfort and spiritual and emotional healing. Continued life is the goal of the first, graceful and meaningful death the goal of the second. If there is to be any dignity and meaning in the death, then a shift to the second goal will become appropriate at some point.

While most people indicate that they wouldn't want to end their lives on a respirator, it must be borne in mind that this journey is never a leap from perfect health to the hospital bed. There will be a thousand perfectly rational and logical decisions between the two. Before your loved one gets on the road that leads to the intensive care unit, explore the map with the physicians and nurses. Ask where the proposed treatment will lead, and don't be satisfied with evasions or "Let's wait and see." As humans, we are inclined to believe that one more treatment, a few more days, will allow us to turn the corner. Just where the road will lead once past the corner is frequently unclear. Knowing the desired destination can make the journey much easier, and the medical staff and your spiritual counselors can help you and your loved one find the right route.

Most of the modern treatments that turn into nightmares

for the dying are perfectly appropriate when the patient is expected to recover. The use of a respirator to get a person through open heart surgery, or past the trauma of an auto accident, is entirely justified. The use of intravenous feeding to rest the digestive system during infection is completely appropriate. What may *not* be appropriate is using these same treatments or painful and invasive diagnostic tests when your loved one is clearly dying of a disease the physicians know they cannot cure. For example, pneumonia has long been known as the "old man's friend." It is a complication that can usher us quickly and relatively easily toward our death when a terminal illness or very advanced age is present. It can be treated with antibiotics and occasionally with a respirator, and your loved one can survive the episode and then later die of another complication, which may be more painful or distressing. Even intravenous fluids are now considered unhelpful in the final few days of life when the body naturally and painlessly dehydrates from lack of interest in fluids, and in fact, this state, called "terminal dehydration," assists the dying by providing chemical changes that reduce pain and anxiety.

Doctors know when they are making real progress and when they are just rearranging the deck chairs on the *Titanic*. Whether you are confronting death or are a caregiver for the dying person, it is important to ask the physician or the nursing staff where you are in the process. Your loved one presumably knows that he has a fatal condition. When the treatment has gone as far as it can go in restoring him to health, the doctor needs to communicate this to him and to the caregivers. Though it is good practice for the dying person to be kept completely informed about his condition, he may not wish to be told the details of what is happening to him. As caregiver, you may decide that the medical professionals are not the appropriate persons to inform him. In those instances, you may have the task of telling your loved one that further therapeutic treatment is not appropriate. This information should be given in the most loving and sensitive way you can manage, as hard as it may be to get the words out.

It is very important for the caregivers and the one who is dying to have made decisions about when and under what circumstances to discontinue curative treatment before a crisis comes and to have discussed them with the physicians and nursing staff. Often the crises that occur and require immediate decision making are difficulty in absorbing and using enough oxygen, an increase in pain or agitation, sudden growth of a tumor that changes life expectancy owing to obstruction of some vital function, or inability to eat or drink liquids. At these or other junctures, the pressure by the staff or the family, or within your own mind, can be overwhelming to *do* something, anything, even if it is the *wrong* thing, which it usually is. Remember, the dying process is an inevitable and largely passive one. Massive intervention at the eleventh hour will only prolong a physically and emotionally painful process. It may eke out a few extra hours or even days of suffering for your loved one, but the end will be no different.

෨ ෨ ෨ ෨ ෨ ෨ ෨ ෨ ෨ ෨ ෨ ෨ ෨ ෨ ෨ ෨ ෨ ෨

David: I was helping care for a young man named Bill, who was thirty years old and dying in the hospital. His had been a long and hard-fought struggle, and he was assisted by a loving and determined family. He had recurrent pneumonia and was on 100 percent oxygen, an ominous sign. He was increasingly mentally confused and frightened.

I left the hospital one night, sure that the next thing they were going to want to do was put an oxygen pressure mask on him. This dreadful device is heavy and noisy and straps tightly around the head so that the oxygen is forced into the lungs under pressure. It prevents the patient from talking to those around him and is very uncomfortable. I had never known a person with a terminal illness to survive with one more than a few days. It was obvious that Bill's time was very short, and the use of this mask would just prolong the inevitable and make it impossible for him to communicate. When I came back to the hospital the next morning, Bill had the pressure mask on.

The next day Bill began to die. His mother and I escaped for a few moments to the waiting room to discuss the treatment options still remaining to her. I said, "You have to decide first whether we are treating Bill to cure him or whether we are treating him to ease his transition."

His mother thought a moment and said, "We have to ease his transition. I need to tell the doctor."

She could at last accept the inevitable, that today was the day Bill was going to die. She reached a level of serenity that I had not seen in her in weeks, despite the enormous psychological and emotional blow that was now coming down on her like a juggernaut.

ﷺ ﷺ ﷺ ﷺ ﷺ ﷺ ﷺ ﷺ ﷺ ﷺ ﷺ ﷺ ﷺ ﷺ ﷺ ﷺ ﷺ ﷺ

When the time we call the active dying stage comes, it is often accompanied by feelings of guilt, in your loved one and his caregivers. The dying person may feel he is giving up, while his caregivers may feel that in some way they are responsible for his death. Try to remember during this difficult time that death is not occurring because anyone is giving up or because you are discontinuing a treatment the physicians are telling you is ineffective. None of the people involved is responsible for this death—the disease is. If you must blame something, blame it. What you and your loved one are doing, as difficult as it may be, is accepting the inevitable and trying your best to make sure that everyone, including him, can find some meaning, comfort, and dignity in his dying.

Assisted Suicide and Euthanasia

Many people with terminal illnesses contemplate suicide. They may think that they will not be able to stand the pain associated with their illness, or they may not want to burden their loved ones with their care during the dying time. Many want their physicians to help them die by giving them an overdose of some drug. These are complicated personal and social issues for which we have no definite answers, only some guidance.

We believe that the dying have a right to their dignity and to be free of pain. Many life-threatening illnesses do not involve a great deal of pain, and very effective means are available for pain management. The dying have a right to make decisions regarding the kind of care they wish to have. Life ultimately belongs to the person living it, but it may be shared by many others. All within the circle of love have a right to have input in any decision that is made regarding an intentional termination of life.

Some, but not all, physicians are willing to help ease a patient over to the other side at the very end, often by increasing the morphine dosage enough to cause respiratory depression, which allows the final breath to come sooner. Again, this is enormously controversial. If this assistance is desired at the end, it needs to be discussed with the doctor. His willingness to help in this way cannot be assumed. The issues surrounding assisted suicide or euthanasia are not only moral, however we may feel about them. Those who actively assist may find themselves facing legal charges, particularly now that the issues have become a matter of public controversy.

It is important to work through all of the questions, personal, moral, and legal. Suicide is not a decision that can be corrected later. It is not a decision that should be taken alone. All of the affected persons need to be consulted, as does any spiritual adviser.

As a caregiver, it is helpful to know that thoughts of suicide in the dying are quite normal. If your loved one brings up the subject, we suggest that you listen carefully to what he is saying. Often the dying need to talk about ending their lives, but most never follow through, even if they have actively made preparations for it. If you think your loved one needs psychological or spiritual help, you may arrange for it if he is willing. The dying time is a time for you to spend together, to increase your intimacy and sharing. The most helpful way to make this most personal of all decisions is in an atmosphere of love and trust.

Rights and Responsibilities ೦೦

Cultivating a good relationship with the attending physician is all-important. It is likely that specialists will be consulted who are unfamiliar to you and who may be unfamiliar with the needs and desires of your loved one. You do not have to deal directly with these doctors if you do not wish to. You may choose to receive any information and recommendations the specialists have through your attending physician. The specialists just need to be informed that that is your wish. Most laypeople have no basis or training by which they can intelligently choose among alternatives presented by the specialists; they need the advice and help of their regular physician before making those choices. The attending physician, if you tell him that this is your wish, can instruct the specialists to communicate with you through him, so that you do not have to face what may be an awkward situation in front of the dying person. If hospital personnel arrive to perform a procedure you have not discussed with the physician, you may refuse to allow it until you have spoken with him. If he is not readily available, you may ask to have him paged. Hospitals are very short staffed now, and it is best to make sure that an error is not being made. These issues should be handled sensitively by all concerned.

Many, if not most, laypeople are intimidated by doctors, especially if the arena where the interaction takes place is the hospital or the doctor's office. Doctors speak in a strange language, they dress in lab coats, and they generally exude a sense of confidence and knowledge that may overwhelm you. What often happens is that you or the person confronting death may feel unable to voice your questions or preferences to the physician. Such feelings are common and can lead to complete paralysis in the caregiving process because of misinformation, miscommunication, and the resulting conflict between the attending medical staff and the dying person and his caregivers.

Physicians and nurses, by and large, are in the healing business because they want to help people. They are completely human, meaning they make mistakes, they can say things that sound insensitive, and they hate delivering bad news to their patients. A common fault of physicians is that they tend to retreat into medical jargon if they are losing a patient to death. As a caregiver or patient, you have the right to ask any question you want and to insist that the doctors not use their professional language, and if they do, you can always ask the nursing staff for a translation. A patient may refuse any particular treatment and may maintain control of his dying. You have the right to expect and demand the highest level of care for your loved one when in the hospital, hospice, or other health care facility and from the home health or hospice nurses if the patient is at home.

At the same time, you have a responsibility to recognize the humanity in the health care providers and to express clearly what it is that you want, either as someone confronting death or as the caregiver, be it a change or discontinuation of treatment, help in the physical care of the dying person, or anything else. Laypeople often simply fall silent, overwhelmed by the drama unfolding before them, and the physicians and nurses have to play a mind-reading game to try to figure out what to do and what is wanted. This is not fair to you, to them, or to your loved one.

Legal and Financial Issues

Several legal issues need to be addressed. Whether the dying person has a last will and testament will be important if he has property that has not been placed in trust or if there are bank accounts or safety deposit boxes that will not be accessible in the event of his death. Consult with an attorney on the best way to handle these issues. If your loved one has no property, then a will may be unnecessary.

If your loved one is in the hospital, he should be provided with the opportunity to execute a living will. Another frequently used legal document is a durable power of attorney for health care. These documents are designed to protect the dying person and his wishes regarding treatment and to provide for who shall have decision-making authority if he cannot exercise it himself. These are complex documents and should not be attempted without legal counsel. If living wills are recognized in your state, the state legislature will usually provide the exact wording for these documents and whether or not they need to be officially recorded. Departure from these legal requirements may invalidate the document.

DURABLE POWER OF ATTORNEY

A durable power of attorney for health care will designate another person, whomever the person executing the document wishes, to make decisions regarding his health care if he is unable to do so. This power is revocable at will but otherwise continues until the maker is deceased. It may make provision for certain persons to be allowed access to the person during his illness. The person designated as attorney should be someone trusted and who has been instructed by the dying person as to his wishes concerning treatment. It need not be a blood relative or spouse.

LIVING WILL

A living will is a different kind of document from the durable power of attorney. It does not hurt to execute both of these documents, but they should not be in conflict regarding their directions for medical treatment. The living will (the form may be available from the hospital) states whether or not the patient wants to have any extraordinary means used to keep him alive, such as a respirator. This document too continues in force until revoked. It is addressed to the hospital and to the dying person's physician and will be a good record of his desires regarding medical treatment.

LAST WILL AND TESTAMENT

A last will and testament is a document that will make provision for the distribution of the property of your loved one after death and may provide for funeral arrangements. It should not be confused with the living will, which addresses only the question of medical treatment.

Many people facing death are reluctant to discuss their will with their loved ones. This reluctance can have many unfortunate consequences. Wills and insurance policies may be misplaced or unavailable. Many people do not understand that a safety deposit box will be sealed at death and the documents within it will be out of reach for some time. For instance, it is common to keep the last will and testament in a safety deposit box. The will is necessary to open the estate and appoint the executor. If the box is sealed at death, there will be no way for the executor to retrieve the will to open the estate. A lengthy period of legal maneuvering will be necessary to rectify this oversight, when it could all be avoided by having the will in the right place at the beginning. The loose ends left at the end of life need to be tidied up as much as possible before the death occurs. This means that all documents needed to file claims and to establish the estate in law need to be immediately available.

Having the will prepared (preferably by a lawyer) and available will give you peace of mind and help to ensure that the wishes of your loved one are known and will be carried out. They are especially important if he lives in a nontraditional family, where the lines of legal authority are unclear or where they run contrary to his wishes. If, for instance, he wants his companion or a friend to have the legal authority to make health care decisions on his behalf instead of his parents or adult children, then that must be provided for in a durable power of attorney. His verbally expressed wish that this be so will not be effective if he is no longer able to express himself.

FINANCES

The dying time lays many financial burdens upon the dying and their caregivers, whether at home or in the hospital. People often feel overwhelmed by the costs and the paperwork required to manage payment of bills to all of the providers of the health care support that is needed. Your hospice or hospital may have a financial counselor and caseworker to assist you in applying for any available public benefits or in filing health insurance forms.

After the death, the estate may require the filing of an income tax return and perhaps an inheritance tax return if the estate is large enough. All the documents necessary for the preparation of these returns will need to be preserved. If you will be acting as the executor of the estate, we urge you to consult with an experienced tax attorney and accountant in the preparation of the returns. If the one facing death is willing, having an estate planner or attorney review the arrangements made in a will may save a great deal of money in taxes by planning the estate properly.

The time when a person is dying is emotionally stressful for his family and direct caregivers, but also for the health care workers. Especially if they have treated him for some time, an emotional bond will have developed between them. Times of great stress are difficult for everybody, and often conflict will develop that otherwise would not. Much of this can be avoided by remembering that it is the person who is dying who is important, no one else. Everyone has a role to play, but the room of a dying person is not the place to resolve other conflicts. The role of the caregiver, whether friend or family or professional, is to assist the loved one in considering and implementing the many choices of the dying time and to ease the coming transition as much as possible.

2 ∽ *A Healing Environment*

A LAST RESORT
I wish there were a place for gracious dying
A high place with a distant view
Where we could gather for a celebration
Of life and death and friendships, old and new.

I'd like a place where there would be good music
Good food and wine—and laughter, games and fun,
And quiet talk with friends, and good discussion
Of what will happen when this life is done. . . .

HELEN ANSLEY AT AGE NINETY

To the One Facing Death ∽

Although this chapter is written to your caregiver, we invite you to read about the many ways you can create a positive and peaceful environment for yourself. We have included ideas from our experiences of observing and helping clients and friends create healing and soothing environments for the awesome transition called dying. We and your caregivers want your environment to be the most comfortable, loving, and supportive place possible for you. Since you've never done this before, consider the ideas that we suggest, and add or subtract some of your own. Remember, this is your time. You can choose.

To the Caregiver ⚭

It is a labor of love to create a safe and peaceful environment in which the transition into spirit will eventually take place. Your love of and communication with the one facing death, your creativity, and the help of friends and relatives will all enhance the process. When in doubt, ask your loved one. She will become an expert on the surrounding environment and its impact on her.

The Importance of Surroundings ⚭

The person who is dying and bedridden lives in a very small physical world. The larger world outside may fade from memory as the room and perhaps the bathroom take on new importance. As surroundings shrink, sensitivities and irritants may loom larger. For example, noise, perfumes, cigarette smoke, discomfort, and the chitchat of well-meaning visitors may become triggers for anger or anxiety. The dying person has the right to live and die as she wishes in dignity and peace. Sometimes this means changing the surroundings or asking visitors to be more sensitive to her particular needs or to the concept that her world is changed and smaller.

Who's in Charge? ⚭

Many dying at home hate the isolation of a back bedroom and really want their sickbed in the living room so that life goes on around them. And others dislike the hubbub of household activity and prefer a quiet atmosphere, especially toward the very end of life. Some enjoy kids and dogs in their bed; others shudder at the thought. To make matters even more confusing for the caregiver, preferences change with the dying just as they do with the living. Flexibility within reason is a healthy goal in this situation. If your loved one requests something unreasonable, it is still okay to say no. As her world becomes smaller, her perspective may get narrower and she may become less communicative. In all of these situations, as in life in general, you cannot be and do all things perfectly.

A Return to the Senses

When your loved one is dying and her world is reduced, she will notice and welcome a return to the simple pleasures of her five senses. These are ways you can provide her with loving stimulation in the hours, days, or weeks before she dies. However, as always, we suggest consulting with her about any big changes before implementing them. If your loved one doesn't want what you suggest, try to let it go without feeling unappreciated.

SEEING

Soft lighting is usually welcome in the sickroom. Fluorescent lighting seems to be the most irritating, both because of the type of light produced and the constant hum of the fixture itself. Unfortunately, fluorescent lights are de rigueur in most hospitals. They may be physically disturbing and may cause headaches with prolonged use. When possible, replace the fluorescent light source with natural light by tilting blinds or using an incandescent lamp. Bulbs softened with pink may be used for added relaxation. Bright lights can be uncomfortable for anyone who is sick. If brighter lights are needed for caregiving or any reason, use them temporarily and then turn them off. Shaded lamps at eye level are more comfortable than overhead lights. This may involve the use of a nightstand at a height appropriate for reaching needed items and low enough for light to be diverted from your loved one's face. Long reaches and hard-to-turn switches may also become inconvenient and frustrating. Remote controls and touch sensors are available for many appliances and electronic devices, such as television, stereo, ceiling fans, and other lights. Using these devices enhances and prolongs your loved one's independence and control.

Nurses have long known and reported decreased depression and accelerated healing in patients whose hospital room faces something alive, such as a tree, lawn, courtyard, or even a sky view. In the home as well, the bed of your loved one can be turned to allow an outdoor view. The next best choice is living plants. The presence of things of the earth is soothing to one who is contemplating her changing circumstances. Flowers are usually enjoyed visually, but check first to see if the fragrance is welcome.

Color is known to be stimulating or soothing, and your loved one may have her own preferences about the colors she prefers in her surroundings. Generally, softer, muted tones are best. The water colors of greens and blues are soothing, as are the colors from the inside of a shell, the peaches and pinks. Off whites and soft beiges are better than stark white. Colors to avoid are red, yellow, orange, and any shades of color that are electric, since they may evoke strong feelings of anxiety.

❁❁❁ ❁❁❁ ❁❁❁ ❁❁❁ ❁❁❁ ❁❁❁ ❁❁❁ ❁❁❁ ❁❁❁ ❁❁❁ ❁❁❁ ❁❁❁ ❁❁❁ ❁❁❁ ❁❁❁ ❁❁❁ ❁❁❁ ❁❁❁

Joan: One delightful and energetic daughter of a client created a wonderful visual gift for her mother. Betsy was a photographer and made the rounds to all of her mother's close friends, supporters, and healing professionals and took five-by-seven photos, with each person holding a big block letter. When developed and assembled on a large colorful poster, the message read "WE LOVE YOU MARTHA." She hung it high enough so that Martha could enjoy it while lying flat in bed. Other clients have done the same for get-well cards, artwork from grandchildren, pictures of the family, friends, and cats, or other memorabilia. Others have enjoyed favorite objects with personal or spiritual meaning strategically placed so that no matter what position they were in, they could enjoy seeing something of meaning and value to them as individuals.

ﾒ ﾒ ﾒ ﾒ ﾒ ﾒ ﾒ ﾒ ﾒ ﾒ ﾒ ﾒ ﾒ ﾒ ﾒ ﾒ ﾒ ﾒ

Much time is spent by the dying one with her eyes closed, although she is awake or in a dreamy state. You may have read about using visualization to help improve the internal visual landscape or, more specifically, to enhance physical, emotional, or spiritual healing. However, many people reach this stage of life without having tried anything like visualization. Guided imagery is a form of visualization, and all it takes is your gentle and familiar voice. Although you may ask a nurse or therapist to make an audiotape of guided imagery for your loved one, you may also read aloud the suggested scripts and directions for their use, which are included at the back of this book. A helpful image for everyone to have is that of a safe place. (See appendix.) You may find that as you read this script to your loved one, your own safe place begins to emerge in your mind as well. Talking about the images perceived by each of you is a lovely way to increase intimacy and sharing at ever deeper levels. Caregivers and the dying who were formerly lovers and are no longer capable of or interested in sexual intimacy can find these to be opportunities for new kinds of intimacy. It may also pave a smoother road to recovery for the caregiver, when being together physically is no longer possible.

HEARING

The dying are often exquisitely aware of sounds around them, though some seem oblivious to a constantly running television. Beeping watches, ringing phones (ringers can be turned off or muffled on most phones), barking dogs, or loud voices may be sources of irritation that you as caregiver may want to screen out.

The sense of hearing is present even when the dying seem to be in a coma, so paying close attention to conversations being held across your loved one is very important. Many survivors of near-death experiences or coma have reported details of disrespectful conversations they overheard. Pay particular attention to discussing bad news of the world or of friends and family. Your loved one has enough to think and worry about with her own life ending. Some visiting and chatter among friends in the presence of your loved one may be welcome and may bring good cheer, but look out for signs of anxiety or irritation. She may not have the emotional or physical strength to set healthy boundaries for herself with people she may be afraid to offend. Sometimes conversations in the sickroom, especially if there are more than one or two visitors, are confusing and exhausting. It is okay to ask visitors to limit their conversation and check their emotional baggage at the door. You and your loved one may decide what she would like to be exposed to in terms of people's problems with their lives or with losing her. If she is feeling drained rather than enhanced by listening to any visitor or any sounds, you and she have the right to end the visit or activity.

Music evokes psychophysiological responses through its effect on the limbic system of the brain. This system contributes to evoking complex and subtle changes in emotional, intellectual, or spiritual states of being. Just ask any parent exposed to heavy metal music! In the preparation time before dying, soothing music is very comforting and helps pass the time. In choosing CDs or tapes for the sickroom, avoid those where a selection suddenly changes tempo, gets spooky or loud, or in any way breaks the mood of peacefulness. Some new age music, some classical music, and carefully selected vocals are our favorite choices. The danger in using vocals is that they often have a theme that might have been attractive in the past but now may be depressing. We have asked clients and caregivers for recommendations of music, and their favorites and ours are included in the appendix.

TOUCHING

We humans need to be touched. For five thousand years of written history and fifteen thousand years of pictorial history on the walls of caves, we have recorded this intimate human experience. The need for babies to be touched is well documented; in fact, they can die or fail to thrive if not touched enough. When facing dying, we need touch more than ever and may be unable to instigate or even ask for it. Sitting and holding your loved one's hand while talking or being silent is a profoundly caring act and makes an enormous difference. A soft stuffed animal or the warmth of a real pet can be sweet sources of touch as well. Beloved pets, sensitive to your loved one's needs, can have an important role here. At this time, the love of a dog or cat is much more relevant than any concern about germs. If dirty, pets, like humans, can be washed. We encourage including a pet in the dying time. Some understanding physicians and nurses even turn their heads the other way when a fuzzy friend is brought to the hospital for a short visit, and enlightened health care facilities openly allow pet visits when approved by the physician.

ⰭⰭⰭ ⰭⰭⰭ ⰭⰭⰭ ⰭⰭⰭ ⰭⰭⰭ ⰭⰭⰭ ⰭⰭⰭ ⰭⰭⰭ ⰭⰭⰭ ⰭⰭⰭ ⰭⰭⰭ ⰭⰭⰭ ⰭⰭⰭ ⰭⰭⰭ ⰭⰭⰭ ⰭⰭⰭ ⰭⰭⰭ ⰭⰭⰭ

David: Evan had been in the hospital for many months. Even though he had wonderful support from family and friends, he missed his dog, Basil, terribly. Basil was a Tibetan spaniel that he had found wandering about at a flea market, and they had become very close. For the longest time we didn't see what we could do about it, hospitals being the antiseptic places they are. Another hospital in town specifically forbade visits by pets.

One day when the doctor was in the room, I mentioned how much Evan missed his Basil. The doctor said, "Well, why don't you bring him up here to the hospital? I'll sign an order allowing the visit if you'll promise me to bathe him before you bring him." We got right on it, and Basil arrived about the time of the evening meal. It made such a difference! Basil hopped up on the bed and buried himself in Evan's arms. He stayed the rest of that night and made many return trips over the ensuing weeks. Evan's morale improved enormously, and he actually felt better after the visits. We were fortunate in being in a hospital that allowed such visits and in being surrounded by health care providers who understood the deep connection between patients and their pets.

ⰭⰭⰭ ⰭⰭⰭ ⰭⰭⰭ ⰭⰭⰭ ⰭⰭⰭ ⰭⰭⰭ ⰭⰭⰭ ⰭⰭⰭ ⰭⰭⰭ ⰭⰭⰭ ⰭⰭⰭ ⰭⰭⰭ ⰭⰭⰭ ⰭⰭⰭ ⰭⰭⰭ ⰭⰭⰭ ⰭⰭⰭ ⰭⰭⰭ

Don't be intimidated by more deliberate forms of touch such as massage. There are numerous benefits to a professional massage.

It reduces feelings of isolation; helps with changed body image; reduces stress, decreases pain and discomfort; stimulates blood and lymphatic circulation; and enhances an awareness of physical boundaries, which is sometimes helpful when one is sick and confused. A professional massage from a licensed or certified (some states do not license) massage therapist is wonderful and can usually be arranged even in a hospital, but a massage from you is a different kind of treat.

Here's a simple approach for you to try. First, ask if this kind of touch is what is wanted and to what specific parts of the body. A full-body massage may feel overwhelming and for some might be painful. Keep the body covered with a sheet, uncovering only the part being massaged. This is to prevent chilling, which happens with relaxation and with the use of lotions. If turning is difficult, your massage may be administered in stages, waiting for the next comfortable time to turn. For a back massage, for example, your loved one may be lying on her side or abdomen. A soothing massage oil, even a light vegetable oil, should be poured into your hands to reach body temperature, rather than drizzled cold onto her back, which is startling. The bottle of oil can also be left in warm water for a few minutes to bring it to a comfortable temperature. Or you may start with a warmed, unscented lotion or add an aromatherapy essential oil, as we describe later in this chapter. Beginning with your hands fully lubricated, take long, smooth strokes across the shoulders and down the back. The muscles across the tops of the shoulders get sore from lying on the side, and gentle kneading massage of these muscles is usually welcome. The long muscles along both sides of the spinal column respond well to long, slow, smooth strokes from top to bottom and bottom to top. Try to avoid lifting your hands once they have made contact, as this gives a smoother massage. Slow and steady rhythmical motion, without sudden jerks or changes in pressure, is best. You may detect knotted muscles in the shoulders and along the spine, and those can be worked out with firm and smooth pressure with the thumbs. Ask at various points if she is comfortable, if more or less pressure is desired, and if she is warm. If she falls asleep, you're probably on the right track! Arms and legs are massaged individually, uncovering only one part at a time. Again, long smooth strokes with well-lubricated hands are the most effective. The amount of desired pressure may vary from place to place. Pay close attention to bony prominences such as tailbone, pelvic bones, knees, and ankles. Very light massage in these areas helps circulation so critical to preventing pressure sores. Try to make it emotionally safe for your loved one to complain if it doesn't feel right. Remember you are both learning this dying process.

If you would like to limit your massage to hands and/or feet, that can bring a unique kind of touch pleasure. Reflexology is an ancient practice of touch of hands, feet, and ears, in which each part is divided into zones. The zones correspond to every part of the body, and massage to those parts relieves pain and increases circulation of blood and energy. A foot reflexology chart is included in the appendix. Slow, gentle massage of the feet and/or hands not only feels wonderful, but has the positive benefits of evoking feelings of wholeness and comfort. A certified reflexologist can be enlisted for this work. You may also try a gentle foot massage yourself, unless your loved one's feet are very sensitive to tickling or she has neuropathy (nerve pain) in her feet.

First, arrange yourself and your loved one comfortably, exposing only the foot or hand to be massaged. Pour massage oil or lotion into your hands to bring it to body temperature. Follow the long lines of the foot or hand in long, smooth, rhythmical strokes. Include the toes and fingers, where nerve endings are plentiful. As with the massage technique just discussed, keep your hands from lifting and coming back, since that can feel disruptive. Your technique isn't what is important; your loving intention behind the effort and the intimate time together are a lovely gift.

Another way to touch is to allow the flow of life energy through you to your loved one. Many describe this as a warmth, a tingling, or a pleasant kind of sensation. After twenty-five years of scientific studies that demonstrate the effectiveness of the energy-based touch therapies, many registered nurses, particularly holistic nurses and hospice nurses, are now educated to provide these therapies and practice various forms of energy healing in hospitals, offices, and home health all over the world. For a professional touch therapy treatment, you can call a nurse who is a Reiki therapist or healing touch practitioner. But know that all people have the power to transmit healing and soothing energy, even if it is not done according to a specific technique. To begin, close your eyes, get quiet inside, and focus all your attention on your loved one and what you are about to do. Relax your body and put your hands on the part of her body that needs attention (pain relief, soothing, etc.). Or you can place them over her heart or at the crown of her head. Imagine the flow of energy (some sense it as light or color) from the crown of your own head down to your heart, where you add your own love, branching it out to your arms, down to your hands, and out to your loved one. It is very likely that she will feel a pleasant warmth even if your hands are cool to touch. Keep your hands in place for as long as you like, perhaps several minutes. This is a wonderful way to administer touch. If actual physical touch is no longer comfortable or pleasant, you may hold your hands an inch or two from the skin and send the energy just as well.

⧉ ⧉ ⧉ ⧉ ⧉ ⧉ ⧉ ⧉ ⧉ ⧉ ⧉ ⧉ ⧉ ⧉ ⧉ ⧉ ⧉ ⧉

Joan: Angie, a ten-year-old girl who was dying from complications of a disease called scleroderma, loved it when I used the nursing touch therapies with her, particularly Reiki. In the hospital during the evening of her death, she was restless and fearful. She was aware that the end of her life was near and was worried about whether she had been good enough to go to heaven. I had been keeping my hands in place over her heart and at the crown of her head and talking with her about safety and peace. She was quiet and occasionally attentive and smiling with my hands in place. I was interrupted from this energy work now and then for the staff to perform a procedure, and she would become restless and fearful again, even though the procedure was not disturbing or painful. Any time I would return my hands to those two places, she would become tranquil again. During one of the interruptions, even though Angie had hardly spoken at all that day, she opened her eyes and said, "Don't stop. That feels good. It feels like the angels are here."

⧉ ⧉ ⧉ ⧉ ⧉ ⧉ ⧉ ⧉ ⧉ ⧉ ⧉ ⧉ ⧉ ⧉ ⧉ ⧉ ⧉ ⧉

For many reasons, a hand over the heart and a hand at the crown of the head feel especially soothing. Those are the areas where we are most easily encouraged to be at peace and to feel spiritually safe when touched during the dying time. Of course, simply holding your loved one's hand in both of yours helps her feel less alone as well.

SMELLING

In the sickroom, smells can become problematic. Good ventilation, a ceiling fan, opening windows to fresh air, some air fresheners, a drop of perfume oil to a cool light bulb before turning on the light, or incense are a few solutions. The odors associated with bed care and some diseases are often more of a problem to outsiders, since the sense of smell exhausts itself fairly quickly. So our focus will be on creating the environment with the positive benefits of aroma, some to cover negative odors, some to simply create positive aromas.

Aromatherapy is a term that was coined in the 1930s, although the practice has been around for thousands of years. The concept is one of healing and soothing with aromatic oils. Essential oils may be purchased in a variety of places: health food stores, spas, metaphysical stores, even some health and beauty shops. Some oils may be expensive, so it is a good idea to try a whiff before you invest in them. Bear in mind, however, that in this form they are very concentrated and strong. These essential oils are nongreasy and are what provide the characteristic fragrance of a flower. You may mix them with oil or lotion for massage; or their aroma may be inhaled by (1) placing a tiny drop at the nostril or upper lip; (2) holding a scented cotton ball or washcloth (wet or dry) close to the nose; (3) adding a few drops in the bath or a bowl of hot water and then breathing the steam. Or they may be dispensed in any number of commercial diffusers or nebulizers, which emit the aroma. Some antiseptic fragrances may seem better suited for the room than on the person. Some people wear essential oil in a specially made hollow pendant so that they can smell it throughout the day.

Aromatherapy is a nontoxic remedy without any side effects. Not all essential oils smell particularly pleasant to everybody, and illness may cause changes in preference, so individual choice continues to be important in smelling as in all of the senses already discussed.

Like listening to music, aromatherapy works by stimulating the limbic system of the brain, where it can contribute to evoking complex and subtle changes in emotional, intellectual, or spiritual states of being. Various essential oils can induce euphoria, spiritual awareness, a sense of peace, or feelings of increased energy or decreased depression. Here are some examples of essential oils recommended by aromatherapists and, more important, by those who are dying and their caregivers.

1. *For relaxing and soothing:* lavender, chamomile, rose, sandalwood, bergamot, eucalyptus (which is also good for respiratory symptoms)
2. *For lifting depression and reducing confusion:* ylang-ylang, rose, clary sage, sandalwood
3. *For pain:* clary sage
4. *For increasing alertness and energy:* clary sage, neroli, rosemary
5. *For nausea:* peppermint, chamomile
6. *For disinfecting and deodorizing:* lavender, tea tree, peppermint, lemon, lemongrass, rose, clove
7. *For spiritual awareness and meditation:* sandalwood, ylang-ylang, frankincense, bergamot, cedarwood, myrrh
8. *For insomnia:* chamomile, lavender

TASTING

A sweet mouth and pleasant tastes are a gift to one who is confined to bed. In terms of enjoying the sense of taste, several ideas have been found helpful in our experience.

Joan: Tracy was in the early phases of the dying time. Because of the many drugs she had taken for her cancer, her sense of taste was nearly gone, and because of the advanced stage of her illness, her appetite was very low. She fully accepted that she was going to die but was interested in eating as well as possible, because she knew that she would feel less weak and queasy if she could eat. Her partner, Rob, brought meals on a tray and would take them away an hour later uneaten. He tried every suggestion he had read to make the tray more attractive: candles, a flower, a colorful napkin, a love note, attractive arrangement of foods. One day, after listening to Rob's frustration, I asked Tracy about this. She confided in me that she felt guilty about asking for meals and not eating them, especially since Rob was going to such effort to entice her. I asked why she couldn't eat. She said, "It is so much. I can't eat it all."

Tracy was overwhelmed by the volume of food and gave up before she started. I suggested to Rob that he serve very tiny portions of whatever she really liked. He said, "Well, that will be crackers and peanut butter." I suggested preparing one cracker with peanut butter and cutting it into four pieces, putting it on a dish on the same beautifully decorated tray and seeing what happened. It worked. He repeated this with tiny servings of anything she liked, and Tracy was able to enjoy her sense of taste again.

⚭ ⚭ ⚭ ⚭ ⚭ ⚭ ⚭ ⚭ ⚭ ⚭ ⚭ ⚭ ⚭ ⚭ ⚭ ⚭ ⚭ ⚭

To a well person, the size of these portions may seem odd, but to someone in Tracy's state, it can be a welcome relief. The same goes for any type of food that sounds appealing to your loved one but isn't eaten when served. Try serving a very small portion on a normal-size plate, and cut it into pieces about half of a normal bite-size piece. With beverages, a small juice glass only half-full will often inspire more liquid intake than a larger glass or even a smaller one that is full.

The temperature of fluids seems important to everyone's sense of taste. This preference can also change unexpectedly when someone feels ill. Ice-cold or very hot drinks may produce intestinal cramping, gas, or hiccups, but room temperature drinks may not. On the other hand, room temperature drinks that are usually enjoyed hot or cold may produce nausea. Your loved one may experience odd cravings or want to confine food choices to one or two foods such as ice cream and Jell-O. Carbonated drinks are troublesome with hiccups and gas, but some find them very desirable. As with aromas, the illness or the medications may drastically change food preferences. Experimenting helps and, as always, when in doubt, ask.

Food left in the environment for too long is often nauseating to a person without an appetite. Even if the food is left uneaten, it is probably better to remove the tray and try again later. The exception would be soft mints or lemon drops to keep the mouth tasting sweet or to freshen the breath when visitors arrive. Water and ice chips at the bedside are a good idea, so the dying person doesn't have to ask for everything so frequently. Straws kept nearby, as well as towels for spills, are essential.

Guidelines for Visitors

If visitors ask what they can do or bring, or if you as the caregiver wish they would, you can suggest that they read this section. You may want to post some of the following on the door to your loved one's room. Add your own ideas to the list as well.

SOME GUIDELINES FOR VISITORS

1. A visitor is anyone who is not one of the primary caregivers.
2. Do not visit without calling ahead unless you have been asked to do so.
3. Ask about a convenient time to arrive, and stick to the schedule.
4. Ask about how long a visit is welcome, and leave promptly. If you are not given a length of time to stay, look for the earliest signs of fatigue and then leave.
5. Offer to give the caregiver a break while you are there.
6. Ask the sick person how she is feeling. Remember that the most supportive thing you can offer is your full attention.
7. Ask the caregiver how she is feeling.
8. Recognize that the sick person's world is very small, perhaps only one room.
9. Don't lie. Gentle diplomacy without dishonesty helps create trust.
10. Check your emotional baggage at the door. A very sick person is not likely to have the strength to hear about your problems.

11. Leave the news of world tragedy outside the room. If she is watching it on TV, use the time to learn what her feelings about it are, not to expound your own.

12. Surround this person with positives rather than negatives. This is not to suggest denying what is happening. Pollyannas and hopelessly moping visitors are both irritating. Honest concern works best.

13. If you love this person, say so. Love heals the soul. And there's magic in the telling.

14. Don't offer unsolicited advice. If you think your idea would be especially helpful, ask if it is wanted.

15. Even if you can stay only a minute, sit down so that you are nearer the eye level of the person in bed. Sitting near the head of the bed and holding her hand make a brief visit seem more meaningful, as opposed to waving from the door.

16. Visit alone rather than with a lot of other friends. The temptation is too great for visitors to talk among themselves and over the bed, and the sick person often feels overwhelmed and left out.

17. If the sick person seems more interested in TV or dozing, ask if she wants you to stay. If she does, stay even if you're not receiving anything from the visit. Sometimes your silent presence with or without touching is all that is necessary.

18. Be willing to listen even to the silence.

19. No moralizing, judging, criticizing, or blaming.

20. Never minimize the person's feelings, as in "You're not thinking about this properly," or "Don't you realize . . ." "You have to stop feeling this way," or "Don't cry/Don't feel bad. . . ." These are ways to protect your feelings, not hers.

21. Don't assume the person wants or is able to recover or does not want to recover, and allow her the dignity of having those feelings without arguing or minimizing the situation with statements such as "Oh, you'll be better in no time. I'll see you on the golf course."

22. A very ill person spends a lot of time thinking about her condition. You can find out if she wants to talk about it by asking.

23. Crying is okay for everybody.

24. Avoid more than two visitors (in addition to caregivers) in the room at one time.

25. If the sick person is entertaining you as a guest, let her know gently that this isn't necessary.

26. Know who is in charge in the sickroom and defer to her judgment.

THINGS VISITORS CAN OFFER TO DO

1. Sign up for a block of caregiving time.

2. Organize friends to bring meals, share overnight care, and send letters.

3. Bring pictures, decorative items, or any supply that is needed.

4. Welcome gifts may include a stuffed animal, a journal, bath powder, music tapes, mints, incense, flowers, rented movies, a gift certificate for a massage for either the sick person or the caregiver.

5. Offer to clean the house, mow the grass, water the house-plants, take the car for service, walk the pets, write the checks, write letters, take the children for outings.

6. Remember your talents: fixing things, singing, crocheting, painting pictures, taking photographs of friends.

7. Hug the caregiver and offer encouragement. Hug the one who is sick, if she is up to it. Hug yourself for caring.
8. When the loved one is gone, offer to help take things home from the facility or return the sickroom to a normal room in the home.

Having considered caring for the senses, as well as creating comfortable surroundings in the room and in the stimulation from people and pets, you can see clearly that a healing environment is much more than a physical space. It is a total environment created for loving and soothing body, mind, and spirit. It is important to pay attention to the details that enhance serenity, dignity, and peace for your loved one's dying time.

3   ✂   *Comfort*

There are no guarantees.
From the viewpoint of fear none are strong enough.
From the viewpoint of love none are necessary.
EMMANUEL

To the One Facing Death   ✂

No one should have to go into their dying time in fear and pain. Most people facing death, even those who are at peace that the end of their life is near, insist that dying, while often very sad, is not what bothers them the most. What they dread is pain, fear about the loss of control, and not knowing what the other side will be like. People who have survived near-death experiences tell us that it is actually wonderful, beautiful, and peaceful. However, since nearly everyone who dies is doing it for the first time in conscious memory, getting from here to there is what most of us worry about. You may encounter pain and fear, but you don't have to endure intense suffering needlessly. Medicine and nursing have advanced to the point where the management of pain and anxiety is considered very important. Talk with your doctor about how aggressively she is willing to provide for your comfort with medications. Talk with your nurse about your expectations that your needs will be met. You are never asking too much when you ask that you be kept comfortable. And if their regimen isn't working, you or your caregiver may demand another, regardless of the day of the week or time of night.

Many people also fear the need for intimate care while they are incapacitated and bedridden. It is not unusual for people to require partial or total bed care during the last days, weeks, or sometimes even months before death comes. In this chapter we discuss comfort measures for the most common needs during this time, such as your care if confined to bed. We include management of nausea, fear, pain, and shortness of breath. You may find it difficult to contemplate having these problems or needing to receive this kind of care, and none of this may turn out to be your experience. However, nearly everyone provides and/or receives physical care at some point during her lifetime. This happens to be your time. Just as giving birth may be hard and almost always requires assistance, dying is hard work for some, and if that includes you, you deserve to receive help in that process.

To the Caregiver

You have chosen to care for a loved one who is facing the end of life. What an awesome responsibility! And what an honor to be included in one of the most intimate journeys anyone can take. Giving care and comfort to a person reaching death is an act of love that will change you forever. Although an entire chapter is devoted to your care during this time, we want to emphasize that you do not have to perform any of these procedures perfectly, on time, or alone. If you find you are striving for perfection or rigid scheduling in caregiving, it is a good idea to let go of that; it always leads to failure. If you find that you insist on doing everything yourself without help, try to figure out your motivation. Resentment and burnout are the natural outcomes of these approaches, and we recommend trying a gentler way. A talk with a supportive friend or therapist may help if you think this is a problem.

Providing Comfort ⌒

Most people really don't feel very well when they are dying. We probably didn't feel good when we were being born, either. And most mothers will admit that they didn't feel very well when giving birth. All of us proceed through two of these processes; and mothers, all three. Although these events are natural and normal, the days of believing nothing can be done about discomfort are over. Medical and nursing care have come a long way. People are now choosing to give birth and to die with varying degrees of alertness or sedation, feeling and pushing through discomfort or enjoying relief from virtually all sensation through the liberal use of medication. People may also change their minds many times along the way. However, provision of comfort is much more than the use of medications and medical procedures. Here we will discuss basic physical care of your loved one. For further information or clarification, your nurse is a good source.

IN BED AT HOME OR IN THE HOSPITAL

When your loved one has reached the stage of being partially or totally confined to bed, rental of a hospital bed is very helpful, and the cost is often covered by health care plans. Linens are smaller, turning is easier, and the beds adjust (usually electrically) to varying heights as well as to relative positions of head, knees, and feet. However, rental of a hospital bed triggers strong emotion in some who are facing death. For some people, leaving their own bed signals giving up and moving into the deathbed. This may be a difficult decision, but we encourage you to consider your comfort in providing care and the comfort of your loved one in receiving it. The decision is a joint one between you and her. Most people adjust to the change because it is so much easier to manage total bed care and find comfort in a hospital bed.

In either home or hospital, we recommend having on hand a good supply of disposable pads for underneath the bottom. This helps avoid linen changes when there is an accident. Smooth, clean sheets and an assortment of pillows help to maintain comfort and good body alignment. Your nurse can show you how to arrange a draw sheet to assist you in turning your loved one if she is no longer able to turn herself. She can also show you how to change linens with your loved one still in the bed. Finally, an egg-crate mattress is a real comfort for those who have lost a lot of weight and now have bony prominences. It is just what it sounds like: a mattress pad shaped like an egg crate, about two inches thick, made of foam rubber. Because of the indentations, the skin can maintain blood and air circulation better, thus preventing bedsores. Other choices include inflatable mattresses that fit on the hospital bed, or alternating pressure devices. These may be purchased at a medical supply company, or your nurse may order whatever devices are helpful.

BODY MECHANICS

Good body mechanics will save your back. When lifting, pulling, bending over, or otherwise using your back in providing care, raise the bed to a comfortable height for you. Bend your knees and use your leg muscles whenever possible to prevent back strain. If your loved one has lost a lot of weight, you may perceive her to be very light, but any adult is heavy and possibly too much to lift with a bent back. Any time you can use your legs and keep a straight back, you will be helping yourself.

Positioning someone in bed comfortably is based on a few principles that are easy to follow. Good body alignment helps maintain comfort, and frequent turning helps prevent bedsores. If your loved one is on her back, a thin pillow under her head and neck will prevent too much neck flexion. Her back should be relatively straight, and if the head of the bed is elevated, her hips should be at about the fold in the bed. Elevating the knees helps prevent her from slipping down toward the foot of the bed. If she slips down, her back and neck will curve uncomfortably. Pillows are helpful for propping up arms or under calves to take pressure off the heels. If she is on her side, the same principles apply, with a thicker pillow under her head to keep her neck in alignment and with pillows between her uppermost arm and her body, between the knees, and between the ankles.

Turning from side to side or back is best done every two to three hours. You may need help with this if your loved one is no longer able to assist you.

Skin Care and Hygiene ⚭

Providing hygienic care to another person offers many unwanted opportunities to spread germs. On the whole, common sense is sufficient to prevent the spread of infection from you to your loved one or from her to you. In general, hand washing before handling food and before and after intimate body contact is all that you need to remember. Disposable latex gloves are essential in the sickroom. If you may be exposed to blood and other body fluids, it is very important that you wear gloves. This protects you from germs and also makes care more pleasant. Contracting illness from caring for a person with a disease spread by exposure to blood and body fluids is preventable with the use of gloves and good hand washing. Wearing a mask is not necessary unless you or your loved one has an illness spread through the air, such as a respiratory infection. Ask your doctor or nurse if this is a concern.

Keeping the skin in good condition is important and one of the biggest challenges of taking care of a person in bed. Pressure sores (also called decubitus ulcers or bedsores) may be avoided by frequent turning and gentle massage; clean, dry linens; relief of pressure; and especially by keeping the skin very clean and dry. Keeping skin clean is important even if total bed care is not required. If your loved one is using a bedside commode or able to go to the toilet, substituting hypoallergenic and flushable wet wipes for toilet paper may be helpful if bowel movements are loose or hemorrhoids are present. If you need to learn how to assist your loved one with a urinal or bedpan, ask your nurse to show you the easiest way to manage.

GIVING A BED BATH

A daily bath is a comfort to both body and mind. Feeling fresh and clean is a simple pleasure you can provide. If you have never given a bed bath before, you will learn through trial and error and will probably make a few messes along the way. Here are some guidelines to get you started.

THINGS TO ASSEMBLE

a large basin with warm water
liquid soap or moisturizing body wash
two or three washcloths (more if there is bowel incontinence)
towels and a light cover or sheet
lotion, cornstarch-based powder, and lip moisturizer

HOW TO DO IT

If movement causes the person pain, plan the bath for thirty to sixty minutes after a dose of pain medication. Try to assure privacy. Begin by exposing only the area to be washed, and cover it with a sheet, towel, or blanket before proceeding to the next area. The direction to be washed is from the face down to the feet, skipping genitals until last. As you soap each area, rinse and dry it thoroughly. Ask your loved one if you are applying the right amount of pressure. She may prefer lotion or powder in various places. Plain powder cakes in moist creases, but cornstarch doesn't. Cornstarch is also good to sprinkle between her skin and the sheet. As you expose and wash her body, look for reddened or sore areas along bony prominences, such as cheekbones, shoulders, elbows, wrists, shoulder blades, pelvic bones, tailbone, hips, knees, ankles, and heels. If you see redness, gently wash, dry, and lightly massage the area with lotion, then report the problem to your nurse.

After you wash her feet, change to fresh water and wash the genitals and buttocks. The genitals should be washed first, from front to back. You may feel uncomfortable with this part of the bath, but it is important to wash these areas daily or whenever soiled to prevent odors, skin breakdown, and growth of bacteria. Wash with soap, rinse, dry thoroughly, and use a moisture barrier cream or lotion, especially if control of urine or stool causes a problem. Of course, with possible exposure to any body fluids, always use disposable gloves for your safety and comfort.

Shampooing the hair is a challenge, and if your loved one isn't mobile enough to lean over a basin or sink, you have a couple of choices. Your nurse can provide a hard plastic shampoo board or inflatable shampoo board. Both fit under the head, and you can use water and shampoo. They have an opening on the side that lets the water flow into a basin or trash can. A commercially available dry shampoo may also be a good choice. Shampooing your loved one's hair is a simple way to provide pleasure. Most people confined to bed complain that dirty hair is uncomfortable and embarrassing. In addition, shaving your loved one is a kindness often appreciated, since it often requires more energy than he wants to exert. An electric razor is quicker, less messy, and less hazardous, unless you are especially good at shaving another person.

Mouth Care 🞮

Most people, even if unable to bathe themselves, prefer to brush their own teeth. However, if your loved one is unable to perform this function, it is an important part of personal hygiene that needs to be continued. Your loved one may have become a mouth breather or may be receiving oxygen during her illness, so her mouth may be dry, with crusty secretions on her teeth, gums, or lips. Since food and debris collect in everybody's teeth and gums, good hygiene helps prevent infections, odors, and breakdown of oral tissues. Mouth care can be done as often as desired, but once or twice a day is minimal. Here's a method for providing mouth care.

THINGS TO ASSEMBLE

soft toothbrush
toothpaste and nonirritating mouthwash
small basin
small towel
cup of water and maybe a straw
lip-protecting ointment

HOW TO DO IT

Raise the head of the bed as much as comfortable and place a towel under the chin. Allow your loved one to brush her teeth as much as she is able, or brush for her. Look for sores on gums or inner tissues of lips and cheeks, and report them to the nurse. Avoid putting the toothbrush near the back of the throat to prevent gagging. If your loved one wears dentures, they should be removed for cleaning, and the gums can be cleaned with a toothbrush or washcloth. If a significant amount of weight loss has occurred, dentures may no longer fit properly and should be left out if they are irritating the tissues. (Many dentists will reline dentures for their regular patients without charge if they are dying.) After rinsing, using mouthwash, and spitting into a basin, wash the lips and apply a lip-protecting cream or ointment.

Commercially available mouth swabs are useful for mouth care if this procedure isn't feasible, such as when your loved one is lying flat or is not able to swallow. Or you may make your own, using cotton swabs lightly dipped in a home remedy of vegetable oil with honey and a little lemon juice. Experiment with the proportions.

Nourishment

Food and love are closely related for many of us. Letting go of the need to get your loved one to eat when she really doesn't want to anymore is one of the supreme challenges for the caregiver. You may have difficulty seeing that a person whose appetite used to be similar to yours is satisfied with one grape or just one bite of a sandwich. While tips on portion size and presentation are included in chapter 2, we emphasize this again here because it may be helpful to realize that your need to feed your loved one may be significantly greater than her need to eat. As the dying process progresses, appetite naturally decreases and finally stops. Getting your loved one to eat more than she wants may feel like a small victory to you but is often perceived by the dying person as a chore she has to do to make you happy.

Your need to feed may be an unconscious ploy to keep your loved one from leaving you, but it won't work, and it only causes frustration, anger, and feeling unappreciated and rejected. We have seen and intervened in many family fights over food. Food carries a great deal of emotional baggage. Encouragement and a gentle approach are healthy, but be aware of your motives and let your loved one choose. Nagging won't help and will make you both miserable.

If possible, share the meal. It's more enjoyable to eat a meal together. Appetite is often better earlier in the day, so breakfast foods may become more important. If pain is a problem, give her medication thirty to sixty minutes before the meal. Keep the head of the bed elevated slightly after eating. This helps digestion. Frequent small meals work best, and high-calorie supplements are available. Liquids should be offered very frequently, and if constipation is a problem, prune juice is helpful.

Problems That May Arise 〜

NAUSEA OR DIFFICULTY SWALLOWING

Unfortunately, nausea is not unusual in the dying time. In addition to being caused by medication, it may be evidence of an electrolyte imbalance, pain, or simply the body's beginning to let go. Several things can be done to help with this problem. First, decrease any unpleasant odors and procedures just before mealtime. Ask for and use pain and nausea medications. Avoid large volumes of food or foods that are spicy, chocolate, citrus fruits, caffeine, or foods associated with being nauseated. If she is nauseated, encourage your loved one to take slow, deep breaths, eat and drink slowly, and change positions slowly. Other helpful hints: a cool washcloth to the head, some essential oil such as peppermint, or small sips of mint tea at room temperature. Some physicians recommend the use of marijuana or its similar pharmaceutical form. People with nausea and loss of appetite report immediate relief of nausea and an increased appetite when this is used.

If your loved one is hungry but has difficulty swallowing, we suggest the following. Provide oral care before meals or offer something sour such as sour candy or lemon to stimulate saliva. Select foods that melt in the mouth, such as pudding, gelatin, yogurt, or soup. Avoid sticky foods such as peanut butter or soft bread. Cold items such as ice chips, ice cream, or sherbet stimulate the swallowing reflex and may be better tolerated than room temperature foods. If she is having trouble swallowing or is very weak, water can be given in a syringe a few drops at a time to prevent choking. A syringe of appropriate size can be provided by your nurse.

FEAR

Fear and anxiety are natural responses to the tremendous changes occurring. Being a good listener is probably the most profoundly helpful skill you can offer. If the fear is caused by unfinished business with people or plans, helping her verbalize it and making plans to finish the work of living and dying are helpful. If the fear is related to spiritual questions, a spiritual helper or clergyperson may be called. Guided imagery or visualization and relaxation exercises are helpful as well, and a visualization script for reducing anxiety is included in the appendix. If necessary, medication may be prescribed to alleviate severe anxiety.

PAIN

Pain or the fear of it are often a part of the dying process. Pain is a subjective experience, meaning the person experiencing it is the only one who knows when, how much, or where the pain is. If your loved one has lived in chronic pain, she may not display the usual signs of pain, which are grimacing, restlessness, moaning or crying sounds, or even increased heart and respiratory rates. Whether your loved one does or does not act as though she is in pain, it is always best to ask.

Encourage your loved one to be honest with you and her doctor and nurse about the amount and severity of pain she is experiencing. We are often struck by the heroic effort by the dying to convince the doctors and nurses that their pain regimen is working, as though it not working would somehow hurt their feelings. Pain is not a sign of failure or weakness, or a sign that the disease is necessarily worsening, or is to be expected and tolerated. Many people believe that pain is a kind of spiritual punishment and must be endured. Some worry that if they accept adequate pain medication early in the process, nothing will work later if it gets worse. And sadly, most worry about becoming addicted. Our experience tells us none of these is true.

Addiction is not a worry when your loved one is in pain. Taking even strong narcotic medications for relief of physical pain, not for emotional reasons, will not produce a drug addiction in a person who is terminally ill. No matter how much medication is required to keep your loved one comfortable, she is not an addict. The best pain control occurs when medications are taken on a regular schedule instead of waiting for the pain to become severe. Waiting sets up a cycle that is harder to control, and regular dosages prevent the peak of pain and anxiety that is so troubling. Nothing is to be gained by waiting. Some narcotics are now available in time release capsules and skin patches. Some are best given by intravenous pump or subcutaneously in steady doses. Patient-controlled analgesia (PCA) is a good option for maintaining personal control over the balance of discomfort and drowsiness. You and your loved one's doctor and nurse can determine the most appropriate method. Now is not the time to be afraid of narcotics. Unfortunately, some doctors and nurses fear addiction themselves and are unaware that their fears are unfounded. If your loved one is suffering because of your health care provider's fear of causing an addiction, you need to become much more insistent, even to the point of getting another doctor or nurse. No one should suffer needlessly at the end of life.

In addition to medication, some other effective pain relief methods include guided imagery or visualization (see appendix), relaxation exercises, listening to nature sounds, watching a funny movie, massage, and heat or cold to the area that hurts. If the pain is not too severe, humor is appropriate. A good belly laugh actually stimulates the body's production of endorphin, our human brand of morphine. Your sensitivity and timing are obviously important in this realm.

SHORTNESS OF BREATH

Shortness of breath, or "air hunger," is often a frightening feeling, and some assistance from caregivers is welcome. During the dying process, breathing may become more difficult, and your presence and your reassuring calmness can be a real help. Breathing in synchrony with her breathing is a helpful way to be with her. Positioning in bed can help as well. Try raising the head of the bed or placing more pillows behind the back or even helping your loved one lean forward to ease the breathing process. A cool mist humidifier in the room, ice chips in the mouth, and wet washcloths to the tongue or lips can help with thick secretions. If these methods are not sufficient, and your loved one is becoming anxious, you or she may choose to ask for oxygen and/or morphine. There are some points to bear in mind when asking for interventions. Whereas oxygen generally decreases the struggle to breathe toward the end of life, high flow rates of oxygen may prolong the dying process. And while morphine decreases anxiety and depresses the physiological urge to breathe, at high doses toward the end of life it may shorten the dying process. In hospitals and hospice care, both are used frequently in a delicate balance that enables the dying person to maintain comfort and control. Participate in the decisions being made by your doctor and nurse about this balance and whether your loved one is experiencing the necessary relief.

Although providing comfort requires considerable "doing" energy as a caregiver, remember that your love, your "being with," is a way to help your loved one make this journey. If she is in a small, dark, fearful place, your love and your presence can be the spark of light that brings comfort. Never underestimate its power.

The day will come when, after harnessing the winds, the tides, and gravitation, we shall harness for God the energies of love. And on that day, for the second time in the history of the world, man will have discovered fire.
TEILHARD DE CHARDIN

4 ∞ *Healing the Spirit*

I am my beloved's, and my beloved is mine.
SONG OF SONGS, 2:16

To the One Facing Death ∞

When you enter the dying time, you may feel very alone. Even though you may have led an active spiritual life, you may feel abandoned and forsaken. You may be a thoroughgoing rationalist in the Western tradition and feel no need to deal with spiritual matters. Whatever your background, facing your own death will confront you with some of the primary questions of existence. Where do we come from, where are we going, and what is our purpose?

This is an opportunity not only to cultivate and, if need be, repair your relationships with your friends and family and all the people you care about, but also, if you are a believer, to acknowledge your relationship with the higher powers in the universe. There are many opinions about what the Ultimate Reality is like, or even if there is such a thing. It has been our experience that in facing death, everyone does it in his own way, and everyone reaches the same state of grace.

While death itself is the rational, universal end of life for each of us, the process of dying itself is not rational. To find meaning in an individual's death requires more than logic, more than thinking. One viewpoint that we have found useful is to relate to the Other in the same way we relate to music. Music, after all, is just an ordered progression of vibrations or tones, yet it can evoke the deepest feelings and fondest memories. Our Higher Self can be related to in that way, purely on an emotional level, without allowing the intellect to get in the way. It is direct and immediate, much like the feelings of love you have for another person. Remember that in the story in the Bible, when God appeared to Moses in the burning bush, He did not say, "I am Oz, the Great and Powerful. Who are you and why are you here?" Instead, according to the biblical record, He described himself in terms of relationships: "I am the God of Abraham, the God of Isaac, and the God of Jacob." That is the usual way that the idea of the Creator is presented throughout the Bible, in terms of emotional relationships to particular people or events.

If you are not a believer, we suggest that you consider this talk of spiritual reality as poetic truth instead of objective truth. If you believe in no God, or if your conception of that reality does not admit miracles or manifestations, then you can view this accumulated wisdom as the stories and sagas that have helped to give comfort to generations of people just like you. Regardless of your beliefs, you stand at the end of a long chain of traditions and insights, gathered by humankind through the millennia of our existence. Search them, for they contain truth.

To the Caregiver ✵

As your loved one approaches his death, many spiritual issues are likely to surface for both of you. Even as he faces death, you, too, will confront your own mortality. This process can be frightening and can be a challenge to accepted religious beliefs. It can also be an opportunity to expand your understanding of your spiritual nature and help him reach peace of soul and mind, by opening to the song of the universe. It is our experience that the time of transition can, and should be, a time of healing and growth for all concerned.

Spirit as a Loving Presence ✵

Religion and spirituality are not the same, although the two are often confused. For example, Zen Buddhists are not religious in our normal usage of that term, because the belief in a transcendent God is not part of their system; yet we could hardly say they are not spiritual. For the purposes of our discussion, let us define religion as a formalized system of beliefs that is accompanied by a tradition of religious practice. This definition is broad enough to include theistic (Christianity, Judaism, Islam, and others) and nontheistic (Buddhism, Taoism) systems. Spirituality, on the other hand, is not the exclusive possession of any one religious tradition, but is common to them all and indeed exists outside of any religion.

Spirituality is the wisdom that you have accumulated in this life. It is your existence in this world and your connection to all living beings. It may or may not involve a belief in existence after death and any reality on the other side. It is what gives meaning and purpose to our lives. Spirituality is a dynamic state that encourages growth and movement toward wholeness and serenity. It is the point at which religion aims, to encourage moral development and transcendent beauty.

In the dying time you are likely to encounter spiritual distress, in which you experience a disruption in the principles that provide comfort and safety, love and connection, to your Higher Self, to life. You may question the meaning of life and death or your formal belief systems. You may feel anger toward God or the universe or whoever or whatever is doing this to you. You may feel abandoned or see your illness as a punishment for things you may or may not have done in your life. Working through these feelings is a way to bring you to a peaceful state.

☒ ☒ ☒ ☒ ☒ ☒ ☒ ☒ ☒ ☒ ☒ ☒ ☒ ☒ ☒ ☒ ☒

David: I was hospitalized several years ago with pneumonia. I had been running a high fever for several weeks and was confined to bed. Finally I began having difficulty breathing, and the doctor admitted me to the hospital, assuming that I had pneumocystis pneumonia, and asked me whether I wanted to be put on a respirator if that should become necessary. Even though I was pretty scared, I told him if he ever did that, I would come back to haunt him!

I have always been religious, ever since childhood. I was surprised, then, when I found that I couldn't pray. I would have thought that *this* was the time, if there ever was one, but I simply couldn't summon the mental energy necessary. I felt alone and abandoned by God. The heavens seemed to echo in their silence. I was very pleased to have people come and pray for me, since I couldn't myself. I guess I felt betrayed by God. After all, I had tried to live right, I had taken care of other people, I loved God and believed we had a good relationship. The thought that He wasn't there for me was overwhelming. I found out later that that feeling is not at all unusual, but I was unprepared for it, and it threw me. Ever since that episode, I have always taken care to ask a sick person if he would like me to pray with him or for him. Some do, some don't, but most appreciate my concern.

ॐ ॐ ॐ ॐ ॐ ॐ ॐ ॐ ॐ ॐ ॐ ॐ ॐ ॐ ॐ ॐ ॐ ॐ

In facing death, both the person dying and his caregivers may find it difficult to sustain a belief in a loving Creator. Everything we know is intimately bound up with life on this physical plane. Why should we have to leave? Why should our loved ones experience such pain? Well, of course, we all have to face death, our own and those of our loved ones. Some serenity can be achieved by realizing that no matter what we do, whether we are young or old, death will come to claim us.

Philosophers and theologians have been debating the whys and wherefores of good and evil for millennia and will, no doubt, continue until the end of time. If our Creator is all-good, all-knowing, and all-loving, then how can evil exist in the world? Why do people get sick? Why is there starvation? Why is there war? And most important, *why is this happening to me?* Both the person facing death and his caregivers feel that their whole world is crashing down around them. And as much as we plead, as hard as we pray, there will probably be no heavenly voice to give us definitive answers this side of the veil.

That doesn't mean that there are no answers to be found or that you cannot feel Spirit move within you and see it moving within others. All of the people engaged in the care and nurturing of a dying person are reflections of the concern and compassion of that same Spirit or Higher Power that is found in everyone. To take a traditional example, in the biblical story of creation, God is pictured as creating humankind in his image. If we are made in the image and likeness of God, then we, too, are divine creatures. Every face you see is a mirror of the Divine. Every hand that touches you, cares for you, is the hand of God.

In many traditions, one of the energy centers of the body, at the crown of the head, is considered to be the place where the soul or spirit actually leaves the body when biological death occurs. The Divine Spirit is thought to be most present during the dying time, as close as your skin, preparing for the soul's liberation from the body and its reuniting with the Divine. We have attended deaths where this Presence and the spirit of the dying person seemed quite palpable to everyone.

In America, Christianity in its many forms and incarnations is the predominant tradition, but there are dozens of others. Even within those traditions, many find that traditional dogma and belief do not speak to them personally or relate to their life experiences. In a scientific, rational age, belief comes hard to many people, but they will often take from one or more traditions that which they find meaningful and discard the rest. Personal spirituality may exist within a tradition or may choose to stand outside it. It may be complex, involving other spiritual beings and beliefs, or it may be very simple, recognizing only the Higher Self that is in everyone. It may or may not include belief in a deity. Established traditions may be thousands of years old while some, like Sikhism or Mormonism, date back only a few hundred years.

Americans are fortunate in that they are able to choose their own spiritual paths. The great English philosopher Bertrand Russell said that people usually practice the religion into which they were born. A moment's reflection will reveal the truth of this statement. We believe what we believe usually because that is what we have been told by someone else, not because we have consciously examined the alternatives and chosen one set of beliefs over another. Some thinkers today have perceived a spiritual awakening in our society, marked both by a substantial upsurge in traditional religious practices and by a willingness to experiment with new ideas and new forms. All religious traditions renew and reinvent themselves from time to time. These renewals go hand in hand with a developing, worldwide spirituality that seeks the commonality in widely different traditions. The great challenge to accepted belief in the last several centuries has been provided by science, and attempts to reconcile what we know to be scientific truth and what we know to be spiritual truth provide the anvil and hammer that will forge our new and developing spirituality.

There are many published stories today about the near-death experience, some of them incorporated into this book and many of them well documented. These commonly have quite similar characteristics: passing through a tunnel toward a bright light; being greeted by deceased friends and relatives; a review of the life just past. Almost everyone who has had such an experience feels enveloped by love and peace. We have no way of proving the truth or falsity of these stories, but many of the people who have reported these experiences have found new contentment and purpose in their lives.

The God of Childhood and Adult Spirituality ⚭

Many, if not most, people spend only a small part of their conscious waking time considering their spiritual lives. The press of day-to-day living, the pursuit of careers, and the raising of children and tending to our relationships keeps most of us firmly anchored in the physical world we know. As traditionally taught belief systems become less and less relevant to our lives, we either fall away from our religion entirely or go through a profound process of rethinking that produces a new, and more useful, interpretation of our spirituality. This is a natural process, part of what it means to become a mature adult. God forbid that we should be as sure of everything at age forty as when we were eighteen!

As a person approaching death, it is natural for you to consider the ultimate questions. Is there a God? Who is God? What relationship do I have or want with this Being, if any? What will the afterlife be like? Does an afterlife even make sense?

What are the ideals of the spiritual state? Let us summarize them as beauty, joy, love, hope, courage, and strength. Even though your body may be going through unwelcome and unattractive changes, beauty remains an ideal of Western culture, and rightly so. But we are not limited to physical manifestations of beauty. The concept of beauty encompasses the physical, the moral, and the spiritual. When we manifest kindness and compassion, we are beautiful, regardless of our physical state. When we achieve a new spiritual insight, we reflect the beauty of that idea. One of the Buddha's most profound insights was that we, and all living beings, are perfect just as we are, lacking nothing. Our aim in life is to realize this truth. This means that we all possess the same degree of beauty, regardless of our physical state.

Joy may seem far away at this time. What joy can be found in death? That depends upon what you seek. Joy can be found in the simple pleasure of eating something delicious, the birth of a grandchild, or achieving reconciliation after a prolonged estrangement. Joy is experienced in a brilliant sunset, a lovely spring day, and the caring touch of a fellow human being. Joy is not complicated.

Love is what all humans seek. It exists on many levels. It can be passionate, intense, and romantic. It is the primary bond between the generations. It can manifest itself as compassion for our fellow creatures and generate the willingness to make major sacrifices, up to and including the loss of life itself.

Hope is what consoles us today and lets us look toward tomorrow. Even though you are facing death, you can hope to meet your physical end with courage and serenity. Hope that your children or grandchildren will do well in the world and find love and happiness. Hope that others will find meaning in your death and that you will be remembered fondly. "Even though I walk through the valley of the shadow of death, You are with me" (Psalm 23). The discovery of hope, where there is no apparent reason, is a stirring of the spirit.

In facing death and the dying time, there may be times when you will feel your courage slipping away, and the faith you have may seem inadequate. These are the moments when simply talking with or listening to your loved ones will go a long way toward restoring your spirit. Meditation may also help to restore your equilibrium.

Strength can be of many kinds—physical, yes, but also moral

and intellectual. We are encouraged by popular films and books to think of great saints as goody-goody types who do not resemble in the least anyone we know. A study of the records will show you that great saints of all traditions were doers who possessed great strength, unconventional in their times. What kind of strength does Mother Teresa possess, to be able to walk the streets of Calcutta day after day and gather the orphans and sick to her heart? What kind of strength does it take for an AIDS caregiver to return to caregiving again and again and face the certain death of his friends? This quality, which moves people to rise beyond themselves, is strength. You will find it in you. It is part of that divine image that we were endowed with at birth. It remains only to be discovered. Remember, in your spiritual quest, that we are already perfect, lacking nothing.

Many people approaching death torture themselves (or are tortured by others) with the prospect of hell. While you probably have your own ideas about an afterlife, you should be aware that every spiritual tradition has a different view of what happens when we die. If your own beliefs are causing you anxiety on this point, then by all means explore other ideas, perhaps with the guidance of your spiritual counselor.

Caregivers are often concerned about the state of the soul of their dying loved one. They may believe that their loved one will face eternal damnation if he doesn't accept their version of religious truth. These concerns and their expression can cause immense suffering for all concerned. After all, the dying person is closer to encountering spiritual reality than any of the people caring for him. Also, an attempt to coerce religious belief amid the trauma surrounding death focuses attention away from the dying person onto the concerns of others. The caregiver's job is to help his loved one as he wants to be helped, not to show him the way. The drama of death is a unique play each and every time. It is the dying person who writes the script. Regardless of the intensity of the beliefs of others, or the depth of concern for the dying person's spiritual well-being, it is not the job of the caregiver to save him. If the dying person is interested in other spiritual beliefs, he will ask about them. When he wants to talk about his own belief system, then it is appropriate to listen with love and compassion. Judgment has no place in the room of the one who is dying.

Both the dying and their caregivers may want to consult clergy of their own faith in resolving their issues surrounding the approaching death. It is important to find clergy who are sympathetic to the situation of the dying person and his loved ones and family. Clerical intervention can resolve many knotty family problems that may seem insoluble to those involved. The health care providers or support organizations will be able to refer you to appropriate clerical or psychological support, if that is your desire.

Human Value and Dignity

Your value as a human spirit is the sum total of all that you have held important in your life. Your love and wisdom, your acts of kindness and compassion, will live on after you. In Jewish tradition, it is required to remember those who have passed on, for if we forget them, it is as if they died again.

Dignity is a state of grace, one achieved when you reflect on your life's achievements. Most people reach the end of their lives knowing that their behavior has not been perfect, that they have achieved perhaps only a few things that they wanted in life. Compared with the dreams and ambitions of the young, what life is not a bit of a disappointment? The secret that the young have not yet discovered is that life must be experienced and that each experience is shaped by all that has gone before and will shape all that comes after. Be kind to yourself. You have achieved everything that you possibly could in this lifetime, given the experiences and circumstances you encountered. It is enough.

DESTINY AND PURPOSE

Destiny or fate is a concept more common to the ancient Greeks and Romans than to modern society, yet it has had a curious persistence in our everyday lives. Destiny is defined as a preordained course in your life, which you may affect but cannot alter to any significant degree. Many people feel that they were born for a specific purpose, a feeling or intuition that may arise very early in life and provide the inspiration for the course a life will take. Do we really believe this? Undoubtedly many do.

Have you fulfilled your destiny, your purpose? You may have discovered your purpose in life only with your diagnosis of a life-threatening disease. This is not uncommon. The diagnosis may have caused you to change your worldview and values or to pursue a different career path. This destiny, this fate, is not something you can figure out rationally. It is a process of intuition, welling up from inside.

ဟ ဟ ဟ ဟ ဟ ဟ ဟ ဟ ဟ ဟ ဟ ဟ ဟ ဟ ဟ ဟ ဟ ဟ ဟ

David: As with many who have grown up in a life of privilege, I had little idea what I wanted to do with my life as I approached adulthood. Attendance at the university gave me no guidance; there were so many things I might do, but I didn't feel strongly called to any of them. Interested, yes, but not called. In common with many young people, I decided on law school by default, there being nothing else that struck my fancy.

I practiced law successfully for nearly ten years before the AIDS epidemic burst upon our community. I wasn't very happy with law as my career, but I endured it while dreaming of the other paths my life might have taken. However, it was my destiny—my fate, if you will—to be caught up in this spiraling tragedy of epidemic disease. I had read articles about AIDS and knew a very few people who had it, but it didn't touch me deeply.

All that changed after reading a *Newsweek* article in 1987 entitled "The Faces of AIDS: One Year in the Epidemic." I came across a story about a young man from Connecticut, also a lawyer, who was quoted as saying, "AIDS isn't my problem any longer. I'm dying. It's your problem now."

The words seemed to leap off the page. I realized then that AIDS was my problem and that I had finally found my purpose in life. It wasn't something I had to think about, or weigh the pros and cons. I just knew. And even though caring for people with AIDS has broken my heart many, many times, I have never doubted for a moment that I was in the right place, doing the right thing. To borrow a metaphor from World War II, I decided that when I got asked "What did you do in the war, Daddy?" I wanted to have something to say.

∞∞∞∞∞∞∞∞∞∞∞∞∞∞∞∞∞∞∞

As you reflect on your life, you will be able to see the things you have done right and those you have done wrong. Remember, in reviewing your life, that the past is past and doesn't exist anymore, except in your memory. It is all right to forgive yourself for the mistakes you have made. Very few people set out deliberately to make a mistake. Everyone has erred, and since we are rational but fallible creatures, it is all right to be gentle with yourself. It is also praiseworthy to acknowledge the successes you have had and to enjoy your achievements. Every life has accomplished something. As long as the breath of life is within you, you have a way of furthering your destiny.

SERENITY

Serenity is more than the absence of misery and turmoil. Serenity can exist in the most trying of circumstances. Serenity is the achievement of inner contentment and trust in the processes of life. It may be discovered through prayer or meditation, and resources on these methods will be found in the appendix. At the approach of death, many people find serenity eluding them, but this state of grace is a habit of mind, not something introduced from the outside. We continually say, "He made me angry," when we know upon reflection that "he" can't cause anger. Only we can make ourselves angry. Only we can give in to fear. And only we can adopt a serene attitude to our lives and our deaths.

Family Issues

It is not uncommon to have conflict within families, sometimes of the most poisonous kind. It may be that you feel incapable of repairing this damage, particularly if you are very ill. Perhaps you are right. However, if you want to make the attempt, if you are willing to accept the possibility of failure and rejection, you should know that help is available. Clergy can be one resource; social workers or other mental health professionals are another. A kind friend or relative may be another resource. You know, better than any other, that this will be the last chance to put things right with those from whom you may be estranged. You can only do what you can do. Even if you fail, you will at least know you tried.

If you are in the role of caregiver, when your loved one is ready to deal with spiritual issues and the issues surrounding his relationships, you may feel you are incapable of giving assistance, particularly if you are not a member of the immediate family. It is a truism that there are no fights more bitter than family fights. Yet as caregiver it is your job to do what you can to ease the dying process for your loved one. There may come a moment when it seems appropriate to ask if there is anyone he would like to talk to. Often there are things that have never been voiced or people he has ignored for years. Just opening a door like this can cause a rush of emotion and an opportunity for reconciliation. If he asks you to be an intermediary with another person, then you can do this, in the most sensitive way, remembering always that this is not your conflict, it is his. If it is not possible to effect a reconciliation, it is not your fault. You may be the one to ask for the intervention of clergy or other professional help, if you feel inadequate to the task involved. Mostly you can listen and be supportive if your loved one needs help on these issues. Remember, there is no right way or wrong way to do this. The dying person will be your guide as to what he needs and the kinds of support he expects.

We have included, in the appendix, spiritual and religious resources that may assist you and guided meditations that we have found useful. People with strong religious beliefs will find their own traditions to be a continuing source of strength and inspiration. Others with a less well-defined or traditional belief system may find that an exploration of these resources will help them experience the rich diversity of spiritual practices that have nourished humankind through centuries of our conscious existence. We invite all of our readers, believers and nonbelievers alike, to find within the well of inspiration their own spiritual truth as they confront the ultimate issues of life and death.

5 ∽ *Caring for the Caregiver*

*It is only with the heart that one can see rightly;
what is essential is invisible to the eye.*

ANTOINE DE SAINT-EXUPÉRY, THE LITTLE PRINCE

To the One Facing Death ∽

Most of this book has been devoted to your care. While your care is by far the most important issue to all concerned, we hope that reading this chapter will be useful for you, too. On the one hand, we discourage you from being a "good patient," the one who never asks for help, who allows her physical needs to go unmet, who suffers in silence. On the other hand, we encourage you to remember that your caregiver is giving a portion of her life to loving you and caring for you. She has made this choice. Since this section is for her, we would like to suggest some ways you can make her job less difficult.

Your caregiver will be experiencing loss, grief, fear, and many changes in mood from day to day. You, too, will encounter strong emotional changes that may make it hard to feel appreciative, but she will welcome your efforts to do so. If you fail to show appreciation for the work necessary to provide care for you, your caregiver may feel like a martyr. And martyrs are angry people! A "Thank you," a "No, thank you," a smile, an "I love you," are simple courtesies you can offer all the way to the end of your life.

Your misdirected anger and guilt may be difficult for your caregiver to handle. Although any anger you feel about your illness and the circumstances involved is justified, try not to let it find her as a target. The guilt you may feel for being sick and requiring care, or for dying and leaving your caregiver, is understandable but unproductive and, in fact, difficult for your caregiver. You have a right to die and to need help while approaching your death. Appreciating your caregiver for helping you with something you really didn't want to happen may be quite a challenge, but it can be done.

To the Caregiver ☜☞

This chapter is dedicated especially to you and your care. Walking with your loved one on the journey to the edge of physical life is stressful, painful, and perhaps one of the most difficult and rewarding adventures you may ever have. It is an honor and privilege to enter the most intimate moments of another's existence, knowing it is a moment of oneness with all that is. It is a walking together to the final destination, where time stands still and expands to allow the ceasing of a heartbeat and the freeing of a spirit. You may wish you could go, too, to end your physical existence and free your spirit. But like a woman who has just given birth after what seems an eternal struggle and has to let go of what has been a part of herself, you will be left behind by the new form of your loved one. You will have to face typical caregivers' questions: "Who will I be without this person?" and "Am I enough?" Learning to find wholeness in the shared experience of caregiving and the unshared experience of living your own life are your challenges. Caring for yourself during this most important work is essential.

Your Emotions and Your Health

WORDS YOU MAY SAY AND HEAR

"Am I losing my mind?" we often hear from caregivers in the throes of the experience. "Will this ever end?" "Why is this happening?" "Where is God?" "I'm scared I'm going to lose her, yet I wish she would just go ahead and die." All of these phrases and more may enter your mind. The ambiguity of the situation may feel so engulfing that you find yourself saying illogical things. The inescapable nature of constant care may cause you to feel angry and resentful and say things you wish you could take back.

Other friends, relatives, and acquaintances may say things to you that are not helpful. Here is a list of comments we have actually overheard. We share this so that you will understand that you are not the only person who has had to deal with misguided attitudes.

1. Don't cry. You'll make yourself sick.
2. See it as a challenge.
3. Cheer up. It's not the end of the world.
4. Time heals everything.

5. I know what you're feeling.
6. It's God's will.
7. She'll be better off dead.
8. You shouldn't feel that way.
9. Be positive. Be brave. Be strong . . . (Be anything so I will feel better.)
10. You should have seen the way poor Anne died. This is nothing.

It may be more helpful to challenge the person immediately rather than to stew about it and cause yourself extra stress. For example, you could say to number one on the list, "Well, I intend to cry as much as I need to. Not crying is more likely to make me sick." Or to number three, "No, I'm not going to cheer up. It is, in fact, the end of my world as I have known it." You may, of course, add other things, some of which might not be printable. People say things like this to relieve themselves of feelings of pain, anxiety, and loss, not to offer you any relief. It is, in fact, a denial of your grief and your humanity to say those things. Accepting it without response may keep the peace, but it won't be your peace.

SHOCK AND DENIAL

By the time you are caring for someone who is dying, you have probably already dealt with the initial stages of anticipatory grieving (grieving before the loss)—that is, shock and denial. There was the initial *"No!"* that you uttered when you first heard the news and during the time you may have spent believing that your loved one would survive even when it became clear that this could not be true. You may repeat these two stages each time there is a significant change in her health; for example, not believing a scan that shows new metastasis or a sudden worsening of her condition. All of these feelings and thought processes are nature's way of caring for us and keeping us from being psychically overloaded. It is perfectly normal.

GUILT

"Gilt is for French furniture," a friend once remarked after swearing off a lifetime of guilt. Guilt is a totally unproductive emotion. In fact, it is said that guilt is anger you think you don't have a right to have. Whatever guilt is, it doesn't feel very good, and sadly, it is almost universally a part of caregiving.

Why would you feel guilty about giving care to your loved one in her time of need? Some feel it when they have to go to work, or leave for a few hours to get a haircut, or just take a break. You may feel guilty for resenting the time, physical stamina, and lost sleep or for experiencing anger, revulsion at the sights, sounds, and smells, or the wish that she would go ahead and die.

Guilt may also arise from a feeling of blame for your loved one's illness; for example, you may have been the smoker who provided passive smoke or the unfaithful spouse who brought home the disease. You may believe you could have insisted that she get preventive health screenings or that she stop self-destructive behaviors. You may believe that you should be the one dying because she is a better person, younger, more religious, or any number of real or imagined attributes. These sources of guilt are just ways in which you are trying to make sense out of something you may never understand, that someone you treasure is dying and leaving you. It may be a challenge to see any redeeming value in her death, but it is impossible to find redeeming value in your guilt.

SELF-FORGIVENESS

If you honestly believe that you are the cause of your loved one's dying, or that you have caused her harm in the past, you may need some professional help surviving this ordeal with as little scarring as possible. In any event, forgiving yourself and making amends to your loved one are essential. If your guilt is based on anything less concrete, talk it over with a trusted friend, counselor, or clergyperson. You probably did not knowingly hurt her, nor do you want to hurt her now. You could not have predicted the twists and turns of her life, and if you could have controlled her to that extent, would you have really wanted to?

We frequently hear reasons not to forgive the self. Some believe that only God can forgive and that forgiving the self is overstepping one's bounds. Some believe that they don't deserve to be forgiven or that if they were forgiven, they would go out and cause the same harm to another. Have another look at these beliefs and see if you can move past them.

We hope that you can find a seed of compassion for yourself, an understanding of what happened, even though you might not choose to behave the same way with the knowledge and experience you have now. Allow that compassion to grow. This is not an excuse, but an understanding of human frailty and a releasing of judgment. In time, when you are ready, try telling yourself "I forgive you" as many times as you need. Some people do this in a mirror, some in a visualization or meditation. See what works for you. For your own healing, it is time for self-forgiveness and letting go of blame and guilt.

ANGER

Anger is a normal and healthy emotion and is a part of the process of anticipatory grieving, meaning the grief that comes when loss is predicted. Anger may be directed at God or Goddess, the doctors and nurses, the circumstances you find yourself in, or your loved one for acting out or not responding the way you would like. She may not fit the movie image of a quiet and grateful loving person dying without fanfare. She may exhibit new personality traits that you don't particularly like. She may become selfish, raging, demanding, and possessive. She may be withdrawn and rude or say hurtful things. Whatever the cause of your anger, it is real and it can feel overwhelming.

How do you know you are angry if you are not one who freely recognizes or expresses anger? Society has ugly names for people who express anger inappropriately, and most of us learned or were taught that the emotion of anger is "bad" and should not be felt if you are "good." So we deny anger to the extent that we actually may not believe we experience it at all. We may mask it by sensing it as depression, self-pity, or sadness. If you do not think you are in touch with your anger, look for the subtle signs, such as clenched teeth, irritability, frustration, short snappy answers, clenched fists, flushing of the neck and shallow breathing while thinking negative thoughts, obsessive thoughts (or actions) about hitting or hurting someone or a pet, inner rehearsals of cursing someone, muttering, overeating, nausea or loss of appetite just after a "polite" confrontation, and feeling martyred.

What can you do with feelings of anger? On the rational side, try to realize that it is the illness that is causing your loved one's behavior changes and the changes in your life, and direct your anger at the illness. But from the perspective of your emotional health, try to find outlets for your anger, such as talking with a friend or the nurse, writing about your anger, or screaming while beating pillows and crying, preferably out of the hearing of the sick person. The only rules here are that you cannot cause harm to yourself or another living thing, and you cannot destroy valuable property. (While exercise or working out are often cited as good ways to handle anger, they don't help you express it; they help reduce the anxiety and tension associated with it and are helpful in that way.) Expressing anger at God or Goddess is acceptable. No one has ever been struck by lightning for doing that. But not expressing anger at all is detrimental to your immune system and therefore to your health in general. Expressing it inappropriately is detrimental to those around you. Therefore, finding a good way to express anger cleanly is your only healthy option.

FEAR

Caregivers report tidal waves of near panic that come over them at unpredictable times, such as cooking a meal or taking a shower. The fear is layered, and it is sometimes hard to separate the layers. As with anger, you can feel overwhelmed and very lonely. Often there is a painful discrepancy between the fear and terror you are feeling and the way you appear to visitors. They may recognize your tremendous competency in providing care, and you may feel like an impostor as a care provider.

Fear is a normal emotion that occurs when we are threatened. That threat can be the worry that you will not know what to do, that you are not competent to manage the situation, that this illness and your role in it is proof of divine punishment for being bad, and that you will not be able to go on living when your loved one is gone. Fear is a feeling of separation, a longing not to be alone in this dark and scary place. It also produces a physiological response. Fear causes surges of adrenaline, part of the fight or flight response. Long ago, this came in handy when the hunter needed to run from the wild animal or the warrior had to defend his life. When taking care of someone who is dear to you, you don't have the opportunity to run or fight, and you may be left feeling stress, anxiety, and loss of control in the form of a fluttering in the solar plexus area, shortness of breath, or a pounding heart.

We recommend two methods of dealing with fear. The first is to talk to a trusted friend, not someone who will tell you not to be afraid or will try to give advice; perhaps someone who has been in a similar situation. Tell your friend that you need someone to listen. Talking about fear takes an edge off it and provides your friends and supporters with a way in which they can feel helpful and loving toward you. Second, when the wave of fear hits, recognize it without judging yourself, and breathe slowly and deeply into your diaphragm or belly. With each inhaling breath say, "Safety and peace," and with exhaling breath, say, "Fear." Your subconscious mind will quickly learn that you are allowing safety and peace to enter and that you are releasing the fear.

SADNESS

There is perhaps nothing sadder than the knowledge that someone you love will soon be leaving and you will never see her again, at least not in this physical form. Many people avoid talking about it for fear that they will lose their minds or that if they start crying, they will never stop. That kind of profound grief doesn't start with the death of your loved one. It begins from the moment you know that she will leave before you do. Elderly people are acutely aware that the longer they live, the more people they know will die. Younger people have generally not had to think about this unless in a war or caught up in the AIDS epidemic or now the onslaught of breast cancer. Many people feel sadness as a physical ache in the area of the heart. Sadness affects body, mind, and spirit.

What can you do with intense sadness? Crying is very helpful if you are capable of crying. Unfortunately many people have been socialized out of crying to the extent that they are no longer able to do that. Fear of not being able to stop once started prevents that expression of sadness for many. But no one ever started crying who didn't stop. It is also appropriate to cry with the one who is dying. If you cannot cry, try talking about your sad feelings with a friend or a nurse. Writing about it can also be very helpful.

Sometimes we don't recognize sadness, because it masquerades as another, more familiar emotion, such as anger. Exploring the layers of emotion is a way to discover what is really going on between you and the dying person. Being sad together about the impending loss is a way to share another intimacy. People who avoid this intimacy during the dying process often regret it later.

ﾚﾒ ﾚﾒ ﾚﾒ ﾚﾒ ﾚﾒ ﾚﾒ ﾚﾒ ﾚﾒ ﾚﾒ ﾚﾒ ﾚﾒ ﾚﾒ ﾚﾒ ﾚﾒ ﾚﾒ ﾚﾒ ﾚﾒ

David: Danny and I had been together for seventeen years and had known for many years that we were HIV-positive. When he started to get really sick, it didn't come as a surprise for either of us.

For a period of about six months, his anger got the better of him, and he took it out on me as the most convenient target. On top of all my increased responsibilities around the house and his care, it seemed impossible to please him. Formerly, he was one of the sweetest, most emotionally stable people I knew. Although we had never talked about our loss of each other, now we found it impossible to get through the day without at least one shouting match.

This was finally resolved a few months before he died. Friends had told him that he was being too hard on me, and then one day, it just became too much. I took down the suitcase and I said, "That's it. I'm leaving. I can't take this anymore!"

I started to throw things in the suitcase, right there in front of him. Then I became so overcome with emotion that I just ran out of the room, went into the living room, and collapsed on the sofa in tears.

In a few minutes he shuffled into the living room and came over and cradled me on his lap. He stroked my hair and said, "Everything is going to be all right. I'm so sorry I hurt you."

I said, "Danny, nothing is ever going to be all right again." After a while, I calmed down and then helped him back to bed. He never yelled at me again.

ﯦﯦ ﯦﯦ ﯦﯦ ﯦﯦ ﯦﯦ ﯦﯦ ﯦﯦ ﯦﯦ ﯦﯦ ﯦﯦ ﯦﯦ ﯦﯦ ﯦﯦ ﯦﯦ ﯦﯦ ﯦﯦ ﯦﯦ ﯦﯦ

In this situation, intimacy was restored when the emotions finally broke through the layers of anger, then sadness and despair. Although not an answer to the intense pain, this opportunity for human connection was a healing one, and everything changed.

If your sadness is turning into depression that is making it impossible to function—for example, you cannot get out of bed, you are becoming indifferent, you are considering suicide—we urge you to report this to your doctor. An antidepressant, though no cure-all for the heartache, may help you continue to function as a caregiver. This is not recommended for long-term use because part of working through your loss is feeling the intense emotions that accompany it. But this may not be the time you can handle it.

Stress and Burnout

Stress kills, and stress is a part of life. In this paradox is interwoven the need to recognize stress and deal with it. Stress is most often defined as emotional pressure or strain caused by a change or something external to yourself. While you cannot control what is happening externally, such as the impending loss of your loved one and her necessary care, you do have some control over your responses to these stressors.

Stress has an immediate and detrimental effect on the body. It occurs when you are encountering something that produces fear or anger, and you cannot or will not respond by "fight or flight." The sympathetic nervous system responds immediately with increased blood pressure and heart and respiratory rates, cooling of the skin, sweating, and changes in many of the body's chemicals. Interleukins, for example—the body's own cancer-fighting chemicals—are decreased instantly with stress. The immune system is put on red alert, waiting for that tiger attack, and after a time of chronic stress it begins to fail to respond. We need our immune system to fight everything bad this world has to offer: bacteria, viruses, fungi, cancers, and so much more. Bereaved people are often prone to sickness, including diagnoses of cancer, arthritis, diabetes, heart attacks, and routine infections.

We cannot emphasize enough that you must help yourself cope with the stress you naturally encounter as a caregiver.

STRESS

These are some ways your body may signal you that you are suffering from stress:

1. Inability to concentrate, becoming forgetful
2. Heart palpitations, increased blood pressure
3. Insomnia or sleeping too much
4. Headache, backache, shoulder tightness
5. Diarrhea, constipation, nausea, vomiting, compulsive eating
6. Panic, shaky hands
7. Cold, sweaty hands or feet
8. Irritability, clenching your jaw, wringing your hands
9. Loss of your sense of humor
10. Obsessive worrying

If you exhibit these symptoms, it is time to pay attention and begin to find ways to handle your stress.

TIPS FOR HANDLING STRESS

1. Stay aware of your thoughts and feelings. You can stop the negative thoughts about your inadequacy in caring for your loved one. Negative thoughts are stressful. If you know that certain caregiving activities cause you stress and that these activities cannot be avoided, try a breathing exercise before and after each activity. Find ways of expressing feelings rather than "stuffing them." Talking, crying, screaming,

beating a pillow, and writing are some ways that work. Always ask yourself, "How do I feel about this?" Feelings are described with one word, such as angry, hurt, scared, sad, lonely. If you answer with, "I feel as though you don't love me," that is a thought, not a feeling. The feeling underneath that thought, for example, might be "hurt," "scared," "lonely," or "unappreciated."

Mentally repeating positive thoughts is much more helpful than the negative self-talk that may fill your mind. Self-critical thoughts are destructive. Try mentally repeating an affirmation or positive belief, such as "This too will pass" or "We are doing a good job here" or "My love is good enough."

2. Stop setting standards of perfection. They always result in failure. Needing to do things perfectly and behavior that is controlling go hand in hand. You cannot create a perfect death or a perfect dying time for your loved one. "One thing at a time, first things first, and nothing perfect" can be your mantra. If a friend or relative comes and tells you what you could be doing better, it is okay to tell her that you do the best you can, almost all of the time. Trying to do it all and do it perfectly may result in your becoming not only very controlling, but what people in the mental health fields refer to as a martyr. If you feel misunderstood, overworked, and unappreciated, chances are you are feeling like a martyr. And it never feels good to be a martyr! Likewise, resist the temptation to judge yourself. Remember, no one has written a rule book with a grading sheet for caregivers. Make up your own rules and make sure no A's are expected.

3. Stay aware of your own needs. Part of the stress of caregiving is the sheer volume of work. You cannot and should not

try to do it alone. You still need an adequate amount of sleep each night. If your loved one requires active care twenty-four hours a day, some outside help is necessary. Friends or relatives can sign up for four- or eight-hour shifts. Often hospice services have nursing assistants who can provide hours of respite. You also need a balanced diet, exercise about three times a week, activities unrelated to caregiving, solitude, and funny movies. A warm bubble bath may help reduce stress. Changing your routine provides a break. Writing things down helps ameliorate the effects of the forgetfulness you may experience. A list of things to tell the doctor or nurse, problems to solve, or groceries to buy will help you feel less scattered.

All this may be easier said than done. At some point you may require more helpers on call, so that you can meet your needs while your loved one continues to receive care. Sometimes the dying become possessive and demand that you be their only caregiver for weeks or months prior to their death. It is okay to say no to that if it goes on for a long time, or if you simply cannot do it, even though that may seem uncaring. However, as her death draws near, your loved one may truly need you by her constantly, and you may find that you don't want to be away at all in case you miss her final moments. These are difficult times for both of you, and we suggest that you balance the care for yourself with the care of the dying person. If you can't find some comfortable balance, your resentment may be yet another source of stress.

4. Be aware of primal thoughts, such as questions and fears about your own mortality and who you will be after your loved one is gone. A crisis such as caring for a loved one who

is dying shakes us to our core and forces us to confront feelings and beliefs we have always taken for granted. Your spiritual health, financial safety, and even basic identity if you are the significant other are issues that are very real and create questions that may be frightening to ask. It is good to acknowledge these thoughts and questions with a trusted friend or ask for a visit from your clergyperson or therapist.

BURNOUT

Burnout is a condition that results from chronic exposure to stress, known as prolonged stress arousal. It is much more than having a very bad day. It is a condition that renders you unable to provide effective care for yourself or anyone else. It includes the chronic display of signs of stress. In addition, you may feel depersonalized, detached and uncaring, numb, or emotionally exhausted. You may lose your perspective and distort reality; for example, you may find that you are angry at people who are not dying. You may believe that you are totally ineffective in your care. Or you may become negligent and disinterested in your loved one's well-being or grow to hate providing care. If you tend to have problems with addictive substances such as alcohol, drugs, food, or cigarettes, you may find yourself imbibing more or overdoing it.

Several things make one more prone to burnout under stressful situations such as this. If your self-esteem is low, you may need reassurance from someone else. Validation may no longer be available from your loved one, or worse, she may be critical of you and your care. If caring for yourself is not something you readily do, you may see your caregiving as your personal mission, letting your own care suffer. If you have trouble setting healthy boundaries, you may burn out quickly. Your loved one's struggle, though it involves you intensely, is not your struggle. No matter how diligent your care, you will not prevent her death. People who feel it is their duty to "change the things they cannot change" may burn out long before care is no longer needed. Other characteristics that could make you more prone to burnout include lack of regard for yourself, so that you read the information about stress and believe that it doesn't apply to you or put off thinking about it until after the "important" work of caregiving is done.

TIPS FOR HANDLING BURNOUT

To address burnout, you may need some professional help. You most certainly need a break. Trying stress reduction ideas will help (see Tips for Handling Stress), but more than that, addressing any of your patterns of unhealthy caregiving is essential. Healthy helping must include the following.

1. Setting realistic goals. You cannot save or rescue the dying person. That is not your task. Each day take a fresh look at the situation. An outing in the sunshine may have worked last week, but today an accomplishment may be watching a whole movie together.
2. Setting healthy boundaries (having a clear sense of what is self and what is other). Taking on her feelings, pain, or illness will not help your loved one feel more loved. You are there to accompany her on her journey, not make the journey for her. When you hear someone down in a hole yelling for help, it is not much use to jump in with her so that the two of you can yell for help more loudly.

3. Allowing time for yourself. Try to remember that you are not only a caregiver, you are a human being with other needs and interests. Allow others to help.

Steps to Healthy Self-Care 〰️

1. Build a good support system. A support group of caregivers or group of friends or family is essential. No one has to go through this alone.
2. Try to compartmentalize enough to allow solitude of thought, feeling, and space. Time alone to regroup helps prepare for more caregiving. When you are alone, scan your body mentally to see where you may be feeling pockets of tension or pain.
3. Meditate daily. Meditation helps keep you physically healthy and mentally and spiritually centered. The physiological state of meditation is similar to that produced by guided imagery. You may try using one of the scripts available in the appendix by reading it into a tape recorder, or try this simple meditative exercise.

Find a comfortable position, either lying down or sitting up with your back supported. Sitting up may help you stay awake when you become relaxed. Make sure you have some privacy. Close your eyes and take a couple of deep, cleansing breaths. Quietly focus on your breathing while relaxing each part of your body. There is no need to change your normal pattern of breathing.

Visualize a relaxing scene such as the gentle roll of waves in the ocean. To enhance your imagination, try listening to taped ocean sounds or soothing music or just enjoy the silence.

Allow your mind to empty. Mentally recite a relaxing phrase or mantra on the inhalation and exhalation to help reduce the chatter of thoughts. One example is "the water rolls in . . . the water rolls out . . ." If you do that for a while and find yourself mentally making out your grocery list, return to the phrase without judging yourself.

Begin with five minutes at a time for a few days. Gradually increase the time to fifteen minutes or more. Fifteen minutes a day is sufficient to produce definite improvement in physical, emotional, and spiritual health.

4. Remember humor. Humor is healing for the human spirit and a distorted perspective. It also increases circulation, stimulates endorphin release (which literally helps you with physical and emotional pain), and improves immunity. Ask a friend to pick up a funny movie for you. Keep a limerick book handy. Try to keep (or find) your sense of humor.

5. Go outside. Regular exercise rejuvenates the body, helps promote cardiovascular health, and reduces stress. Mentally and physically connecting with what is outdoors helps us stay centered. For example, walk on the ground sometimes instead of concrete to connect with the earth; sit by the water or watch a drizzling rain; notice the fire of the sun and its reflected light on the moon; feel the breeze on your skin; notice the birds, squirrels, or butterflies. Nature provides a connection with the eternal.

6. Maintain your regular interests, even if to a lesser degree. Talk about something other than your loved one. Read something unrelated to illness. Find time for play, creativity, and hobbies.

7. Keep a journal. Studies show that people who write in a journal every day, even for ten minutes, have a healthier immune system. More than a chronicle of the day's events, make it a haven for expressing your deepest feelings. If you are worried about someone reading it, write it on loose paper and discard it. However, you may find later that you are glad to have this record of your story. Photographs may be helpful as well.

8. Remember to breathe. Occasional deep breathing helps reduce stress, and a very deep breath, deep enough to stretch out the diaphragm, signals the body to relax. This is also a good time to scan your body for pockets of tension or pain.

9. Eat well. Remember your nutrition is the fuel that keeps you going. The food pyramid designed by the U.S. Departments of Agriculture and Health and Human Services has replaced the four food groups used since most of us were in school. To follow these recommendations, imagine the bottom of the pyramid with the most space being the recommendation for carbohydrates such as bread, cereal, rice, and pasta (six to eleven servings per day). As the pyramid narrows, imagine listing vegetables (three to five servings per day) and fruit (two to four servings per day). Farther up are the milk, yogurt, and cheese group (two to three servings per day) and the meat, poultry, fish, dry beans, eggs, and nuts group (two to three servings per day). At the apex is the fats, oils, and sweets group (use sparingly). In addition to a healthy balanced diet, people under stress may need more vitamin B-complex and vitamin C. Two food supplements that quickly stimulate the immune system are echinacea and goldenseal. For any of these supplements, follow

label directions. In addition, sixty-four ounces (eight cups) of clean water a day keeps the body well hydrated. Distilled, purified drinking water is preferred.

10. Find ways to be touched. Hugs are fun and therapeutic for most people, but in addition we need touch. Make time for an occasional massage or other touch therapy treatment from a professional.

11. Nourish your spirit. Caregivers often tell us that reading the Serenity Prayer helps them stay focused on themselves and their own well-being while caught up in the dying time of the one they love. Whatever method you choose to nourish your spirit, make sure you do it often.

THE SERENITY PRAYER
God grant me the serenity to accept the things I cannot change,
the courage to change the things I can,
and the wisdom to know the difference.
REINHOLD NIEBUHR

6 ✿ *Changes: Your Body and Mind*

Turn up your light. For even if you don't know where you are going, it will be brighter when you get there.

LAZARIS

To the One Facing Death   ✿

Finding out that your life is ending causes profound changes in you physically, emotionally, mentally, socially, and spiritually. It is helpful to be aware of the nature of these changes.

To the Caregiver   ✿

During the dying time you will watch, sometimes participate, and occasionally rebel against your loved one's physical and emotional transformation. At the end of this chapter we will address your responses to the changes your loved one is encountering during the dying time. Included are tips for understanding and responding helpfully to specific changes in her feelings and behavior.

Grieving for the Future
You Won't Have

For most of us, a future is something we have always taken for granted. We assume we will live to be a particular age, often based on the ages of our parents or grandparents when they died or some internal belief or script about the timing and circumstances of our own death. Some people envision being quite old, and those already on in years may envision being even older. Some always thought they would die young but when faced with death still feel the shock and disbelief that characterize the first stage of grief.

Grief is a condition that affects all human beings and even some animals. It occurs when one has lost or is losing someone or something of inestimable value. Your future is being lost, and that is very significant. Life without a future is inconceivable and confusing to us as humans and can also be quite frightening. Unlike pregnancy, which has a reasonably predictable term, the timing of death is not nearly so certain. When a physician tells you that you have four months to live, she is simply giving you a statistical forecast. You are an individual, and your life and death are your own individual experience. You can trust that your death will occur and that this will happen at the right time.

However, you may know inside that your dying time is upon you, whether it is a matter of weeks or months remaining. Accepting the loss of your future may catapult you into wildly fluctuating emotions and dynamic changes in how you see yourself as the human being and human spirit that you are.

STAGES OF GRIEVING

The stages of grieving have been described by many authors, the first of whom was Elisabeth Kübler-Ross, M.D., in 1969. (See the appendix for readings on dying and bereavement.) What we have learned since then is that these stages can occur simultaneously, in any order and at any time, and that they sometimes change from one hour to the next. Grieving the loss of your future is called anticipatory grief, meaning that your grief is present before your death actually occurs. For you this is the only experienced grief, since after your death the rest of the grief work will fall squarely on your loved ones.

SHOCK AND DENIAL

If you were in complete shock and denial about your condition, you probably would not be reading this book. Denial, however, may be revisited in smaller ways as you find yourself thinking from day to day that all this is not really happening or that if you isolate yourself and stop talking about what is happening, it will all go away. Just as you cannot stare into a bright noonday sun, you may not be able to stare your death in the face consistently. However, it isn't so hard to sit transfixed by a beautiful sunset and be engrossed in its beauty and wonder. As you move closer to your final act, spending time with it won't be a burden, nor will it necessarily be frightening.

ANGER

Another stage of the grieving process is anger. Anger may be a comfortable and familiar emotion for you, but for most people it is a forbidden emotion. Women are often taught that anger is something "ladies" don't express, and if they do, the world has a special name reserved just for them! Men can fear anger, too, seeing it as a loss of control and somehow beneath them. You may find yourself in the dying time without any real life experience that tells you how to feel and express your anger in a healthy way that doesn't wreak havoc on everyone around you.

Why anger? "Why is this happening to me?" "Why did I have to catch this disease?" "Why doesn't some horrible person have this instead of me?" "I'm not old enough. This isn't fair!" are some of the questions and thoughts that provoke strong feelings of anger. They are entirely justified, and so is your anger. It isn't much consolation to hear that everyone is going to die. What is happening is that you are losing your life as you knew it, losing your future, and leaving people you may not want to leave. If that doesn't make you angry, we don't know what would. Anger at God/Goddess/Higher Self is not unusual at this time, and talking with an understanding clergyperson or friend about it may be very helpful.

Your anger may manifest as general grouchiness or full-blown rage at seemingly irrelevant incidents. It may appear as envy of a friend whose body is strong and healthy or still attractive when yours is no longer so. You may feel resentment at the health care establishment, abandonment by friends, or discrimination against a "socially unacceptable" cause of death. Your life's activities are being interrupted, perhaps very prematurely, and your anger at that is normal. (The concept of interrupting your life prematurely is very subjective, as we know quite elderly people in the dying time who want more time to live and feel that life is ending prematurely.)

BARGAINING

In this stage, you may find yourself trying to bargain with God or Goddess—that is, to change who you are or what you do or say in order to appease whom you see to be a punishing deity. You may have thoughts such as "If I stop cursing, I'll go to heaven" or "If I 'become heterosexual' and renounce my lifestyle, and go to church every Sunday, I'll be healthy again." Bargaining is often associated with trying to find some way to remain in control and to postpone what seems to be inevitable.

Clearly, attempting to bargain can also be associated with guilt. All of us have childhood and even societally induced images of how a "good" person should look or act. The "child" part of us may believe that illness and dying are punishment and if we could just figure out how to be "good," all the pain and fear would go away. We would be rewarded with a longer life. When the bargain is struck, a sense of relief ensues temporarily, but rather than helping for very long, the realization that this thinking is pointless may catapult you into depression. Bargaining is as inevitable a part of the dying time as depression, regardless of how well this time is choreographed.

DEPRESSION

Depression is another stage of grieving, perhaps the one most people associate with grieving. Depression is necessary to prepare you for separation from the physical world. You may experience two different kinds of depression in the dying time. The first is called reactive depression—that is, you are reacting with appropriate sadness to losses that have already occurred. Later in this chapter we will discuss changes in your body, for example. The loss of control over those physical changes may trigger acute feelings of profound sadness and depression.

The second kind of depression, which you may find more difficult to share with your caregivers, is the anticipatory depression of impending loss. For example, the loss of the dream of retiring and going fishing or the awareness of the loss of future are impending losses. This anticipatory depression is an introspective sadness that helps you prepare to leave. In this stage you may find yourself not wanting to talk, but preferring to touch or to visit quietly. It is time to probe and to respect your need for introspection.

ACCEPTANCE

Acceptance is described as the final stage in the grieving process. Unfortunately, with modern medicine always trying to prevent death, people often equate acceptance with foolishly giving up too soon. Many die struggling to beat their cause of death. Acceptance of mortality is something that is rarely discussed, much less manifested, particularly in most Western cultures. And although we encourage people with life-threatening disease to fight with every method they find workable, we also encourage everyone, even those who are not sick, to embrace their own mortality. Accepting death as a normal part of life makes fighting disease and stopping the fight equally valid and honorable efforts.

While others may perceive you as withdrawn or having lost all hope, you may find yourself thinking of death as a welcome next step. The stage of acceptance is not one of giving up in despair, but a final peacemaking and willingness to move on to dance the last dance of life. This is an intensely private affair, and you may have little need to relate your thoughts or feelings to others as you enter into a quiet peacefulness.

Acceptance doesn't necessarily make your death occur right away. Often, even those who fully accept that they are dying have a goal to reach before the final transition.

Joan: Richard was a twenty-nine-year-old man I cared for for several years who had a chronic debilitating illness. He felt sick all the time and struggled to keep working because he loved what he did. In September of that year, after another hospitalization and fifth brush with death, he was in my office discussing how many more life-threatening situations he might survive. He knew and accepted that he was going to die of his disease but wondered why he hadn't so far and when it would eventually happen.

I asked him, "What do you want?"

He answered, "I want to be thirty."

I got up from my chair under the rather silly pretense of looking up his birthday on his chart and took some deep breaths to keep from sobbing in front of my patient and now friend; then I said, "Well, Richard, your thirtieth birthday seems to be coming up on November twenty-ninth. I think you can be thirty if that is what you want."

Richard entered the hospital with another infection on November 26. He was very quiet and withdrawn—in fact, disinterested in people and events going on around him. I left town for the Thanksgiving holiday, aware that his birthday would occur over the weekend. I arrived back in town on November 30 to find that Richard had just died quietly, surrounded by his family and friends.

☙ ☙ ☙ ☙ ☙ ☙ ☙ ☙ ☙ ☙ ☙ ☙ ☙ ☙ ☙ ☙ ☙ ☙

We have also known the dying to wait until a favorite holiday or anticipated trip. Or they may die before the winter holiday season, if it was historically a depressing time for them. Men often die before a birthday, and women after. One friend defied all predictions of his imminent death when he found out his first grandchild was due in eight months. He lived long enough to hold his granddaughter and even to see her smile.

Contemplating the fact that you will not have a chance to grow old can be hard, but we hope you will allow yourself the time and freedom to find a way to feel this and release it. As a forty-year-old-man with AIDS once said, "Grumpy old man is a role I've prepared for all my life, and I'm not going to get to play it." However, the future is any time beyond the present. As long as anticipating tomorrow is part of your life, you are continuing to have a future, however brief.

The Signs of a Failing Body ☙

With the passage of time, your physical body will change, sometimes dramatically. If the dying time lasts for a period of months, your body is likely to respond less and less to curative measures. Some of the physical changes you may experience include weight loss, muscle weakness, loss of appetite, loss of stamina, growth of tumors if they are present, weakness in skin integrity, loss of libido or sexual functioning, and perhaps other unexpected changes in the size, shape, or configuration of your body. These changes will be unwelcome, and you may suffer considerable distress at the loss of your former physical appearance and functioning.

CHANGES IN APPEARANCE

Not all dying people change dramatically in appearance, but most do. It is natural to feel distressed by these changes. Friends and family may tell you that your physical appearance isn't what is important, but that your spirit and the love around you are. Your body is the same beloved body (albeit with constant changeover of cells) you have had since birth. It has contained your spirit and your mind, it has transported you anywhere you wanted to go, and it has provided you with the pleasure of all of your senses, including the ability to communicate verbally, physically, and sexually with other human beings. Your body has been and continues to be precious, and watching the gradual deterioration of it is difficult, sometimes even shocking.

Joan: Jimmy was a long-term patient who had always had a bit of a weight problem. Toward the end of his life, I visited him in his home. He was unaware of how much weight he had lost from the effects of his cancer. While I was sitting with him, he happened to look down at his thigh and with an expression of horror cried out, "Is that my leg? It can't be. I've never seen the bones in my leg before." Later, after asking for a mirror to survey the changes in his face and processing his shock and sadness at what he saw, he mused, "Well, I guess I finally found the perfect weight-loss program. But I don't recommend it to anybody. This is the pits."

Having strong feelings about the changes in your physical appearance is normal. Your caregivers may be quite accustomed to your new appearance and are simply grateful to have you present, but that doesn't negate your private feelings of loss. Some people face their dying time feeling such shame at the physical changes that they isolate themselves. Some are so ashamed of not looking good that their embarrassment drives them to keep friends and supporters away. Physical changes are also a constant visual reminder of illness, and if the illness itself carries social stigma, such as AIDS does today, the changes are, in the words of a client, "a big banner announcing my illness to the world."

🙞 🙞 🙞 🙞 🙞 🙞 🙞 🙞 🙞 🙞 🙞 🙞 🙞 🙞 🙞 🙞 🙞

Joan: Alli was a woman in her late forties who lived alone and voiced clearly that she had never wanted to marry or have children. Alli's ovarian cancer had metastasized throughout her abdomen and although she was dying, she felt reasonably well. She had always been very sociable, and until some dramatic physical changes occurred, she was out with friends and working every day.

However, over a period of a couple of months, what had been a mild swelling of her abdomen grew to what appeared to be a seven-month pregnancy. Her straight dark hair had grown back gray and curly after chemotherapy, and, as she remarked, she looked like a menopausal woman having a baby. Alli was terribly embarrassed by this and couldn't see anything positive about the fact that she still felt quite well, enough to keep functioning in the world. She was so embarrassed at questions about her "pregnancy" that she soon isolated herself, even refusing phone calls. She stopped going out and refused visitors for the last six months of her life. Alli died alone and bitter, unable to reconcile herself to the loss of her body as she had known it.

ॐ ॐ ॐ ॐ ॐ ॐ ॐ ॐ ॐ ॐ ॐ ॐ ॐ ॐ ॐ ॐ ॐ ॐ

CHANGES IN FUNCTION

Perhaps just as distressing is the loss of physical function that some experience. Not everyone is bedridden for more than hours or days prior to their death. Although you may envision weeks of living in bed, you may actually continue being up and around until the very end. Some people are able to do that, and obviously that is preferable. But even if that is the case, you are likely to experience loss of the stamina you once enjoyed, and you may find that other changes in function occur as well. The loss of the physical ability to relate to another sexually can be very distressing; likewise, loss of sexual desire can cause conflict and sadness in both the one dying and her sexual partner. Even if this occurs in your body, remember that physical intimacy is still important. Warm caresses, hugs and kisses, and holding hands aren't a replacement for more passionate sexual communication, but they go a long way toward keeping the closeness alive.

Intimate care of your body by another person is discussed in chapter 3. This is a subject that you may find very uncomfortable, if not impossible, to contemplate. But when you are dying, you have the right to receive care, and your responsibility to yourself is to receive it. If that includes allowing others to manage your comfort and bodily functions, then, sadly, you may have to adjust to that change. Dignity at this time for you may include the respectful care of your body's functions. Your job is to allow yourself to receive that care with dignity.

The Signs of a Healing Mind ∽

Your mind is more than your brain or your ability to think. It is the part of you that remembers, thinks, feels, perceives, reminisces, desires comfort and human contact, plans, and creates. The dying time, though profoundly influencing the well-being of your body, also propels your mind into changes that you have no real way of preparing for, at least in Western culture. In other cultures, where death is acknowledged as a normal part of life, even children are prepared for the ultimate and inevitable calling of death at the end of physical existence. You may not have had the opportunity of considering the approach of the end of your life from an emotional or even intellectual standpoint until now. This is overwhelming for most people, and rather than being taken by surprise, we suggest that you acknowledge this monumental phase in the life cycle for what it is: a time beyond which you will never be the same, but in some way will most certainly continue to be.

REDEFINING HEALING,
LETTING GO OF CURING

Healing is a journey toward wholeness. It is an opening to what has been closed or forgotten. It is learning to acknowledge your divinity, embracing the fear and dread, and trusting the forces of life to get you where you need to go. It is learning to love and accept yourself unconditionally. Quite a tall order! It is no wonder we are given a lifetime to learn to heal ourselves. In the dying time you may (and we suggest that you do) continue your healing.

Emotional healing is therefore possible even when your body is clearly failing. Your continued development as a human being leads to wholeness. Here are some ways that clients and friends have moved toward healing the mind during the dying time.

SEVEN WAYS TO HEAL THE MIND

1. Continue and/or develop the aliveness of your mind. Take the time and have the courage to feel honest feelings that accompany the grieving process you are experiencing. Think of new interpretations and perceptions of things you took for granted before. Keep reading or, if vision is a problem, get books on tape, watch or listen to educational programming on TV or radio. Don't retire from life before you have to.

2. Reconnect with what is natural. If possible, go outside in the sunshine and walk or sit in such a way that you have contact, even if only visual, with things of the earth. View water outdoors if available, or as you bathe or drink water, take a moment to appreciate the water and its service to your body. Most of your body and the earth's body is composed of water. When you are outdoors, sense the breeze on your face, or if you are confined to a bed, take a moment to do some deep or rhythmical breathing. Appreciate the breath of life.

3. Allow your senses to come alive and stay alive. As twenty-nine-year-old Richard you met earlier in this chapter once said, "Now that I am dying, I'm noticing that the sky is bluer." Others have learned to appreciate textures such as bark, leaves, flower petals, fabric, or a child's hair. Listen to the subtleties in music or the perfect quiet of stillness.

4. Creativity and productivity don't have to stop. If you continue learning and inspiring yourself and others, you still have an aliveness. You might have lost the physical ability to paint or write, for example, but you can still use your imagination. Even writing in a journal for yourself or creating your legacy for others are creative and productive. Lift the limitations that say you must continue paid work or former activities in order to be productive.

5. Redefine obligations. If you aren't living your life, you're living someone else's. Do only what you choose to do. Talk only to those you want to talk to. Finish responsibilities as you are able, but don't take on any more that you do not consciously desire.

6. Recognize and honor that your perspective will naturally become narrower and narrower. However, try to maintain an interest in making key decisions that affect your comfort and well-being.

7. Stop negative talk about yourself, self-criticism, and judgments. Forgive yourself for your imperfections and mistakes in life. You may not have always done the best you could. But you did the best, given the circumstances and emotional and spiritual health you had at the time. You are forgivable for absolutely everything. If you find this suggestion hard to believe, try talking with a counselor, friend, or clergyperson. It is important.

REVIEWING YOUR LIFE

Reviewing your life is a natural component of healing and moving through this time. You may not have considered your life as a unit of spirit and humanity. Many people think about their lives only from day to day, relive painful mistakes from the past, or anticipate an unrealistic future they can't seem to meet. Now is the time to review your life as a whole—in other words, your place in the great scheme of things. You may find yourself worrying that you will be forgotten or that your existence may not have meaning and significance.

Writing your life's story is a productive way to review your life. This may be in the form of a notebook that you tear out and discard pages from each day if you are reviewing aspects of your life that you don't want to share. Or you may ask some well-intentioned visitor who asks what they can get for you to buy you an attractively bound journal. This is a wonderful way to record what you would like remembered and to create your legacy in writing.

Another possibility is to write letters to all of the people in your life who are significant, to whom you want to be kept dear. These letters can be composed over time and will be treasured gifts after your death.

Technology can provide a more sophisticated means of communication. Some people have had a friend or professional create a videotape of themselves talking to all those who will be left behind. Although some have chosen to use these videos at their own memorial service, most prefer them to be more private and made specifically for their close friends and family. Making two or more videos is also a possibility to encompass all of your objectives.

Some like audiotapes, as the voice may seem preferable or sufficient in creating the memories or messages. Of course, still photography is always useful. However, if your appearance has changed considerably, you may find yourself becoming camera shy. It is your humanity and your spirit that will come through in pictures or videos. Your appearance, though perhaps changed from when you were healthy, will still be welcome to your loved ones.

Unfinished Business ☞

Making peace within yourself and your relationships are the pieces of unfinished business that haunt many people. Ideally these issues are resolved during the healthy years, but you may be facing them now for the first time.

RESPONSIBILITY OR BLAME

You may believe that your life, your illness, and the timing of your dying are events that picked you randomly and that all of this is just bad luck. Or you may have an intuition that your illness and dying are not random and that there is meaning and purpose in life, illness, and death; that you are responsible for it and responsible for learning its messages.

There is a big difference between responsibility and blame for your illness, your dying, or any of the circumstances of your life. As we alluded to in Seven Ways to Heal the Mind earlier, you may have made some choices that you would have done differently if you had known then what you know now. Taking responsibility for having made those choices without judging yourself as a terrible person is healthy. Blaming yourself for having the disease that is causing the end of your life is unproductive. Yes, stress, depression, and unsafe and unhealthy lifestyle choices do lead to death. But so does life. Forgive yourself. You are not to blame for the twists and turns your body is taking. You may simply acknowledge all choices and respond to the consequences. No matter what choices anyone makes, all of us will die.

RELATIONSHIPS

"At least I know who loves me" are words we hear from friends and patients at this time. Relationships in this time become divided into friends and acquaintances. Friends and certain family members will come through and be there for you. Some who you thought were in that category will become quietly absent. This can be very hurtful if you had expectations that these particular people would be your supporters. This is not an uncommon problem experienced by the dying. What is also experienced is the unexpected outpouring of support and help from surprising sources. Try to receive and accept help and love from every source, and release the desire to change those from whom you expected results. Letting go of this resentment can only help you.

However, the relationship issues most likely to trouble you are those that have unfinished business or in which you don't feel valued.

ﻹﻹﻹ ﻹﻹﻹ ﻹﻹﻹ ﻹﻹﻹ ﻹﻹﻹ ﻹﻹﻹ ﻹﻹﻹ ﻹﻹﻹ ﻹﻹﻹ ﻹﻹﻹ ﻹﻹﻹ ﻹﻹﻹ ﻹﻹﻹ ﻹﻹﻹ ﻹﻹﻹ ﻹﻹﻹ ﻹﻹﻹ ﻹﻹﻹ

Joan: Stan, who had been born with multiple deformities and had undergone a lifetime of painful surgeries, was caring for his beautiful younger sister, who was dying of AIDS. Maggie had never been accepted by her family because of her lifestyle and their particular religious beliefs. She was bedridden, and Stan was trying his best to provide for her physical care. Stan usually acted very efficiently, a bit cold, and although he never said anything negative, he had an angry edge to his voice.

Maggie was too sick to do much more than receive care. She talked with me about how difficult his quiet hostility was but couldn't see any choice but to tolerate it.

One day, in his exhaustion, Stan blurted out, "At least you could have taken care of me. I didn't ask for what's wrong with my body." With his own shortened life expectancy, Stan apparently had counted on Maggie's being there to help him when he might need her later. In fact, the whole family had planned for Maggie to be her brother's caregiver when his dying time came.

While Maggie might have been devastated by this remark, she felt a peculiar relief that finally Stan had said what she knew he and the rest of the family were thinking. They fought and argued and cried, fought some more, and finally came to a peaceful resolution with each other, their love winning out over their antagonism for each other's values. Stan later told me that he had not stopped blaming her for her illness, but he decided to stop punishing her for it. Acceptance of Maggie's value and dignity as a human being would have been the next healthy step, but this was as far as this family could go in healing.

☙☙☙ ☙☙☙ ☙☙☙ ☙☙☙ ☙☙☙ ☙☙☙ ☙☙☙ ☙☙☙ ☙☙☙ ☙☙☙ ☙☙☙ ☙☙☙ ☙☙☙ ☙☙☙ ☙☙☙ ☙☙☙ ☙☙☙ ☙☙☙

Releasing the hold that old relationship issues may have on you is part of the work of this time. We suggest that you decide what you want and how you would like to approach the person, and go ahead. Finishing business may include making amends for your former actions or inactions or asking forgiveness, or it may be just the opposite, in which you want an apology, acceptance of you as a person, or just to put an old disagreement to rest. Doing this emotional work internally is very helpful and may be the only opportunity you have if the person is not available. Releasing the past is a necessary part of moving on in peace.

Living with a Loved One's Changes ᛌᛜᛞ

RESPONSES TO STAGES OF GRIEVING FOR THE LOST FUTURE

You as caregiver will also pass through stages of grieving your loved one's impending death. Each stage (and as we said, they may all be apparent on the same day) is difficult to watch and help with, or even endure in its own way. If she is showing signs of denial and isolation, you may find yourself buying into false hope that she will recover. Since many caregivers also experience denial, discerning reality from wishful thinking is a complex process. We suggest that you not try to pry open the doors of denial or judge your loved one, but allow her this normal process unless important decisions need to be made with her consent. It is helpful during this time to be fully present as she reviews her life and tries to become clear about its meaning and purpose. The last days or weeks of life are a time when things can become clear to the dying person. Listening without judgment is a great gift.

Anger is quite difficult for caregivers to endure, especially if your loved one is spewing it all over you and anyone else who comes into the room. Often she may blast anger at the ones she loves the most and may be exceedingly polite to visitors. This may cause you considerable anger as well. The standard advice for dealing with this random anger is to not take it personally, to listen, to allow her as much control as she wants and permit her to ventilate.

All that being said, how do you live with it? You will get your feelings hurt, and hurling hurt back isn't helpful, nor will you feel anything short of guilt about it, even if it does stop the barrage. We never advise accepting abusive behavior, even from the dying. If the anger is overwhelming, leave the room after saying, "I love you. I'll be back later." This is effective, even if difficult, and it is not unkind.

Depression is hard to be around, too, especially when you are feeling it also. Trying to cheer up your loved one when she is depressed about losses that are occurring, such as her strength, or have occurred, such as loss of employment, may be helpful. However, depression about the anticipated loss of a future is best approached quietly with a listening attitude or simply with touch.

Perhaps the stage of acceptance, with its inherent withdrawal, is the hardest for caregivers. In this stage your loved one becomes much more interested in turning toward her future out of her body and much less attuned to you or to anything you do or say. She may face the wall and not respond to you even though you know she is awake and responding to visitors because she is attempting to be polite. Her failure to respond to you may feel like rejection just as you are becoming aware of how precious your remaining time together is. Unfortunately for you, your loved one needs this introspective time to gather up the loose ends of life and prepare to go. Your presence may or may not even be noticed.

RESPONSES TO THE PHYSICAL CHANGES

You may hear yourself in the quiet corners of your mind saying that you are terrible and shallow for grieving the loss of your loved one's physical appearance, functioning (or sexual contact if she has been your partner). Give yourself the emotional space to grieve over this. Although her mind and spirit are what is real and essential, you have also loved and known her physical form as it was in health.

Talking about the changes and your feelings of sadness may help clear the air and open each of you to greater intimacy without all the unspoken wonderings about still feeling attractive and loved. If your loved one was not a sexual partner, it is still important to acknowledge that you both know that her appearance has changed. If she has been a sexual partner, we suggest that you openly acknowledge the loss of sexual intimacy and talk about other ways to feel closeness. Your loved one, even though possibly feeling asexual, will probably welcome the conversation and appreciate knowing that you still want that closeness in spite of the loss of the former physical beauty.

CHANGES THAT SIGNAL A PROBLEM

Sometimes because of illness or medications, your loved one may exhibit personality changes that are difficult or require medical attention. Caregivers often report bitterness, jealousy, irritability, fear, stubbornness, selfishness, and indifference. However, changes that you probably need to report to your nurse include the following, as they may signify a need for a medication change:

1. Unresponsive depression.
2. Unreasonably quick-tempered extremes of sarcasm, abusive anger and bitterness, or physically abusive actions to herself or others.
3. Mental vagueness when usually responsive.
4. Irresponsibility for important financial, physical, or emotional decisions when still capable of responsibility.

5. Planning suicide.
6. Lack of response to important issues or areas of deep interest.
7. Extremes of anxiety, jitters, or restlessness.
8. Paranoid statements or actions.
9. Hallucinations. This can manifest as hearing or seeing frightening things that are not present. This should not be confused with what many dying persons describe to be spiritual visitors (departed relatives and friends). Of concern would be disturbing visual or auditory images, not those that are clearly bringing spiritual peace.

Finally, as you reflect on the metamorphosis of your loved one during the dying time, we offer the comfort of these ancient words from the Upanishads:

From the unreal lead us to the Real,
From darkness lead us to Light.
From death lead us to immortality.

7 ✂ *The Last Dance*

Now cracks a noble heart. Good night, sweet prince,
And flights of angels sing thee to thy rest!
WILLIAM SHAKESPEARE, HAMLET, *Act V, Scene ii*

To the One Facing Death   ✂

This chapter deals solely with what we term the active dying phase of the dying time. While you may know better than anyone when your body begins entering this phase, it is not uncommon for you and your caregivers to need assistance at this time in sorting out the physical, emotional, and spiritual issues that are about to reach their ultimate resolution for you. For many facing their death, this chapter may be difficult to read, yet others will reach an understanding of the process of physical death, and it will help dispel the mystery of the unknown.

To the Caregiver ⟡

If your loved one has been ill for some time, the contemplation of his actual death may seem more than you can bear. The intensity of the caregiving experience, especially if extended over many months, becomes an end in itself. It may seem that death will never come to release your loved one from his suffering. While this denial will help protect your psyche during the period of illness, the end will inevitably approach. This chapter will acquaint you with the details of the physical act of dying so that you may understand the process as it happens. It is our hope, when your loved one has died, that you will be able to look back on the experience and know that you provided good and loving care and that he has successfully made his transition.

No Dress Rehearsal ⟡

In a very strange, paradoxical way, the person with terminal illness and his caregivers are working at cross-purposes as the illness progresses. The one facing death may look forward to the end of the process, while the caregiver is naturally bending every effort to postpone, delay, and avoid it. Neither of these attitudes is wrong or unusual, though it is common for people to feel that "no one (or no good person) should have the feelings I am feeling."

⟡ ⟡ ⟡ ⟡ ⟡ ⟡ ⟡ ⟡ ⟡ ⟡ ⟡ ⟡ ⟡ ⟡ ⟡ ⟡ ⟡ ⟡

David: As I acquired experience in caring for the terminally ill, I found that during the course of the illness I would imagine what the final scene, the death, would be like. I would imagine all of the details, what was happening, who was there, how I would feel. Because of these imaginings, I felt terrible pangs of guilt. These were my friends, and I was conjuring up their deaths!

When one friend was dying, his whole family was gathered around his bed. In her grief, his mother said, "As many times as I have imagined what this would be like, I never got it quite right."

I heard that, and a huge weight rolled off my back. I wasn't the only one who had these feelings and anticipated grief by previewing the loss in imagination. I realized I wasn't a bad person because I had these thoughts, only human. Once I discovered how ordinary I was, and began to talk with other caregivers about these things, I found out that many other people had had the same experience. Negative mind-talk affects everyone, and it can be emotionally crippling for the caregiver.

ॐ ॐ ॐ ॐ ॐ ॐ ॐ ॐ ॐ ॐ ॐ ॐ ॐ ॐ ॐ ॐ ॐ ॐ

As the life of your loved one moves toward its conclusion, you may have conflicting emotions. The terrible pain of anticipating his loss, of imagining what life will be like without him, may be counterbalanced by your wish to have this terrible drama reach its final act. It is not unusual to say to yourself, "If only he would die!" Your life has been forced into this unnatural cycle of caring and waiting, unable to change the outcome, dreading the outcome, but at the same time longing for your life to return to a semblance of normal. As the caregiver, your life is not your own, and this can quite naturally lead to feelings of oppression and being trapped. At the same time, you begin to contemplate your own mortality. You may wonder whether, when your time comes, you will be able to approach your death with the kind of equanimity you are trying to achieve for your loved one. You may ask yourself, if it is your spouse who is dying, who will take care of you in your hour of need. All of these thoughts, while normal and natural, can be unsettling.

On the other hand, if you are the one confronting your own death, you are naturally wondering what will happen to you: "What will death feel like?" Through the months of your illness, you may have contemplated the ultimate questions of existence, but as the active dying process begins, the ideas you have had may seem inadequate. As your body begins to let go, you may find your ability to communicate with others declines. The journey you are embarking on is both the longest and the shortest trip you can make. Your destination is as close as your next breath, yet it seems so far away.

Welcoming the Transition

Once the active dying process has begun, arrange the room as you have discussed with your loved one or as seems comfortable to him. If you have not discussed these matters, then try to play the music that you know he likes. If possible, give him a bed bath, paying close attention to cleaning his face and, if possible, his mouth. Make sure the bed has clean, fresh-smelling sheets. Adjust the lighting to a low level, since intense light can be irritating. Most important, even though you may be in emotional turmoil, try to maintain a sense of calm and spiritual quiet. Some of the breathing or meditative exercises in chapter 5, or guided imagery in the appendix, may be helpful for both of you. The expression of your emotions at this time—crying, holding your loved one, rubbing his back—are all good and appropriate. He needs to know that you love him. As your loved one prepares to leave this world, try to make a peaceful and serene transition for him your goal.

For your loved one, the time of dying is a passive one. Throughout the last days, weeks, or months, he has been preparing himself and those he cares about for his coming transition. In a very real sense, all of your preparations, all of your care, has led up to this day. His body is giving out, and his soul is about to spring free into eternity. This is a time of great grief for you, because once he has gone, you will not experience him in this form again. At the same time, the suffering of the physical body will cease, and he will be free.

Things to Do and Say

How one enters the active phase of dying varies widely. Some enter with full mental clarity, knowing that they are about to depart. More frequently, the slide into active dying will be accompanied by diminished awareness or confusion. The amount of pain medication in use may play a significant role in how lucid your loved one may be. Some people want to be fully aware, while others prefer to be sedated. These are some of the preferences that would be useful for you as caregiver to know before your loved one enters the transition phase.

This may be the moment to say good-bye. Even if he seems to be in a coma, most authorities believe that he can still hear you. Hearing is the last of the senses to go. It is important that he not depart before you have said all that you need to say. If necessary, ask other people to leave the sickroom so that you can have privacy. If there are a number of people who want to exercise this privilege, close friends or family, then you can arrange for each of them to spend a private time with him, in a way that he will not find too exhausting.

ﭏﭏ ﭏﭏ ﭏﭏ ﭏﭏ ﭏﭏ ﭏﭏ ﭏﭏ ﭏﭏ ﭏﭏ ﭏﭏ ﭏﭏ ﭏﭏ ﭏﭏ ﭏﭏ ﭏﭏ ﭏﭏ ﭏﭏ

David: Before Danny, my life partner of seventeen years, had entered his active dying phase, I thought for months that I needed to tell him what a wonderful life he had given me and how much I loved him. I wanted to tell him, but it seemed as though it would be saying good-bye, and I didn't have the courage to get the words out. He had been bedridden for almost eighteen months, and giving care in that situation becomes your life. It seems that it will never end, that this is just the way life is going to be forever.

Well, of course, it doesn't work out that way. When Danny declined to the point that he was clearly dying, I thought I had missed my opportunity to tell him.

The day before he died, he was receiving a lot of Demerol to control his pain. He had ceased speaking and was generally in a semicomatose state. I was sitting next to his bed, and we were alone. All of a sudden, I looked up at him, and he was peering intently at me, with a fully aware look on his face. I decided that it was now or never, and choking with emotion, I sat down on the edge of the bed, took his hand, and said, "My love, I want you to know that you have given meaning and purpose to my life. You have never been more loved than you are at this moment. I will be okay; I know that you can't help leaving me now. It has been the greatest honor to be loved by you. Know that I love you. I always will."

All the time I was speaking, he had a look of the most intense concentration on his face, his eyes never moving from mine. He then got this gentle smile on his face, his body relaxed, and he closed his eyes and went back to sleep. I am so glad

I had that opportunity, at the very end, to express my love and gratitude for the central relationship of my life.

⋈ ⋈ ⋈ ⋈ ⋈ ⋈ ⋈ ⋈ ⋈ ⋈ ⋈ ⋈ ⋈ ⋈ ⋈ ⋈ ⋈ ⋈

One of the things that we have observed, common to almost all deaths, is that the dying person needs the permission of his loved ones to make the transition in a state of peace. Just as the urge to sleep can be overwhelming in healthy people, so the urge to die can become irresistible at the end. Giving permission to your loved one does not hasten the death, it simply makes it emotionally easier. The dying person may ask for permission, but even if he is no longer conscious, it is appropriate to tell him that you will be all right; it is okay for him to go.

⋈ ⋈ ⋈ ⋈ ⋈ ⋈ ⋈ ⋈ ⋈ ⋈ ⋈ ⋈ ⋈ ⋈ ⋈ ⋈ ⋈ ⋈

David: My friend Lynn, a young architect only thirty years old, had been suffering terribly from meningitis for nine months. I had gone to the hospital to relieve his mother, who had been there for three days. In the early evening Lynn had a terrible seizure, and his nurse told me that she didn't think he would live through the night. I called his mother, who lived nearly fifty miles away, and told her to come back to the hospital. After that, I found a nurse's aide to help me give Lynn a bath, and I picked up the room, put his favorite music on, and turned down the lights. I was sitting on the side of the bed crying when Lynn woke up from his seizure. He asked me what was wrong, and all I could manage was, "The doctor says you're not doing too well." He told me to get up in the bed with him, which I had done many times to hold him and rub his back.

This time, though, he wanted to hold me. He put his arms around me and said, "There's nothing to be afraid of. Everything is going to be all right."

When his mom and dad and brother arrived, I took his mother out in the hall, and I said, "Sometime tonight he's going to ask you for permission to die. You have to be able to tell him it's all right." She looked at me, this woman who had never shed a tear openly all during these nine months of struggle, and nodded.

Later that night, around two o'clock in the morning, after another of his seizures, Lynn looked up at his mother and said, "Mom, I can't do this anymore."

She said, "It's all right, honey. You don't have to. It's all right for you to go. I love you."

Lynn relaxed visibly, and even though the seizures continued through the night, the sense of struggle was gone. What was going to happen was going to happen, but he no longer had to fight it. He died in peace with the dawn of the new day.

ता ता ता ता ता ता ता ता ता ता ता ता ता ता ता ता ता ता

The important thing to convey to your loved one, as he is making his transition, is that you love him and that it is all right for him to go, that you will be all right. Many of the dying are reluctant to leave for fear their loved ones will not be able to manage without them. Death is not a failure! You have been preparing for this moment, and your loved one needs to know that you are with him every step of this journey and that you are ready for him to assume his new life and be free of his suffering. He will appreciate your love and your courage in facing his death with him.

The Signs of Impending Death ∞

As the active dying phase progresses, there will be noticeable changes in your loved one's body that you should be aware of, so that you will not be frightened by them and so that you will know when death is imminent. Not all of these symptoms may occur, and they may not happen in this order.

One of the most visible signs of decline will be in the respirations of your loved one. Irregular breathing patterns are quite common, as a result of decreasing blood circulation and the buildup of chemical wastes in the body. Like coaching a woman in labor, the caregiver can synchronize his breathing with the one who is dying to provide comfort and intimacy. Closer to the very end, you may notice a breathing pattern that is called "Cheyne-Stokes" (pronounced "chain stokes"). It is characterized by a struggling for breath and then a ten- to thirty-second period in which no breathing may occur. This pattern may continue for hours or even days. You may hear the term "apnea" being used by the health care providers. This is simply a cessation of breathing for any amount of time. In the later stages, mucus in the mouth may accumulate in the back of the throat, making a distinct sound when your loved one breathes. This is the so-called death rattle, but in many cases it does not occur.

Your loved one may fall asleep for increasing periods and may be difficult to rouse. When he is awake, he may be confused and may not recognize those around him. He may be restless, picking at the bed linens. His arms and legs may draw up into a fetal position. His need for food and drink may cease, as the body seeks to conserve the energy needed for eating. Even though intravenous fluids are no longer appropriate except to administer pain medication, you should always make sure that water or other fluids are available for your loved one if he wants them.

Your loved one's body elimination will usually cease. If a catheter is being used, the urine produced may become much darker and decrease in amount. It is possible that he may lose control of his bladder and bowels, but it is more likely that these problems will decrease as he approaches death.

Another common sign is a deterioration in the strength of the heartbeat, resulting in decreased circulation. Quite typically, the pulse will begin to race hours before death occurs as the heart tries to overcome the buildup of fluids in the lungs. At the same time, the blood pressure will begin to drop, until both pressure and pulse are no longer discernible in his arms and legs. His extremities may begin to feel cool to the touch, and the skin on his arms and legs may deepen in color and become mottled or splotchy.

If your loved one is awake, his vision may become dim or blurred, but his hearing will usually remain very clear until the end. Even if he has been comatose or unresponsive, he may have a sudden moment of clarity. He may open his eyes or stare intensely at something only he can see, or he may rise up in the bed. If you ask what he is seeing, he may tell you that he sees the angels, a beautiful light, or deceased friends and family. He may smile radiantly. This is a good time to hold him and tell him how much you love him and that he should go with the angels. Physical touch is nearly always desired at the end, but if he does not want it, you may envelop him in an invisible blanket of love as though you were touching him. This seems to enhance a sense of calm.

Your loved one may exhibit any or all of these symptoms. The appearance of one does not necessarily herald others.

ⁱⁿ ⁱⁿ ⁱⁿ ⁱⁿ ⁱⁿ ⁱⁿ ⁱⁿ ⁱⁿ ⁱⁿ ⁱⁿ ⁱⁿ ⁱⁿ ⁱⁿ ⁱⁿ ⁱⁿ ⁱⁿ ⁱⁿ ⁱⁿ

David: When my friend Fred was dying, I kept my hand on his heart. Most people, particularly people who don't have a lot of experience at this sort of thing, concentrate on the breath as the sign of life. The problem is that you can't really tell what is going on just by focusing on the breath.

I knew he was near the end. I couldn't get a pulse at his wrist or ankles, and he hadn't had any measurable blood pressure for almost twelve hours. His heartbeat, which had been racing, had fallen and was getting slower and slower. Finally I felt a sharp "thump" under my hand, and he was gone. Many times the heart just gets fainter and fainter and then stops, but his was quite definite. One last sharp beat, and it was over.

ⁱⁿ ⁱⁿ ⁱⁿ ⁱⁿ ⁱⁿ ⁱⁿ ⁱⁿ ⁱⁿ ⁱⁿ ⁱⁿ ⁱⁿ ⁱⁿ ⁱⁿ ⁱⁿ ⁱⁿ ⁱⁿ ⁱⁿ ⁱⁿ

Making Room for the Angels

As your loved one dies, it is important that you "make room for the angels." As you have brought him to the door of death, you need to make mental and spiritual space in your own mind for those beings who we can imagine will be welcoming him on the other side of that door.

If you have had no experience in attending someone's death, it is not unusual for you to have a sensation of panic as the life force subsides. People have been known to scream at or shake the dying person in an effort to arouse him. They will often be successful, but the natural dying rhythm will be interrupted only temporarily. It is important that the dying take place in an atmosphere of peace, calm, and quiet. This will enable your loved one to make his transition in a state of tranquillity and enable his spirit to depart without the emotional burden of deathbed trauma.

٭٭٭ ٭٭٭ ٭٭٭ ٭٭٭ ٭٭٭ ٭٭٭ ٭٭٭ ٭٭٭ ٭٭٭ ٭٭٭ ٭٭٭ ٭٭٭ ٭٭٭ ٭٭٭ ٭٭٭ ٭٭٭ ٭٭٭ ٭٭٭

Joan: Liz fought her cancer valiantly for many months that included chemotherapy and a bone-marrow transplant. She had been willing to endure any treatment anyone suggested. Her children were young, and she didn't want to leave her husband, Mark, who had been such a loving support. Liz, who never believed she would die, was in the hospital trying to treat shortness of breath, hoping along with her doctors that her symptoms were caused by pneumonia. Then her oncologist told her that her cancer had metastasized to her lungs and that her time was very limited, a day or so at the most.

This was the first time Liz acknowledged that she was going to die. She was very frightened about the terrible air hunger that she was feeling, and her doctor told her that he could give her morphine, but that it might hasten her end. She asked him to give her the morphine when she requested it and then called me to the hospital.

When I arrived there was pandemonium. Mark and Liz were both frightened, and friends and relatives were in the room crying. The change from denial to acceptance on Liz's part had happened so suddenly that everyone, including Liz, was near panic. Her denial had helped her fight her disease for as long as she did but prevented her from really addressing her dying.

I took Mark out of the room to a quiet place and said, "Mark, it looks as though Liz is going to be leaving us very soon."

His eyes grew wide with fear and he said, "Do you really think so?" I think he had counted on me to assure him that this was just another temporary setback.

I suggested to him that he have someone get the children and bring them to the hospital and that he clear the hospital room and say whatever he needed to say to Liz. I advised him to give Liz permission to leave him and let her know she would not be forgotten.

Mark immediately assigned a friend to bring the children and then cleared casual visitors from the room. He then went to Liz, crawled into bed with her, and told her things only Liz and the angels heard.

When the children arrived, Liz reminded them that she would always love them and asked them to remember the fun times before the illness changed everything. They hugged and kissed and cried. Then Liz had the children taken out of the room, and I assigned a relative to take care of their needs.

By this time, Liz's breathing had become very labored. She asked for the morphine, and Mark got into bed with her again, held her head in the crook of his arm, kissed her, and talked to her until her breathing became gentler, easier, and then finally stopped. All of her loved ones were standing around her bed holding hands. As Liz's spirit lifted, everything in the room seemed lighter and everyone's pain seemed easier. They all experienced it and talked about it months later, saying that each could feel her kind presence as though meant only for them.

You, too, have need of the ministering angels. We seem to feel their presence as death occurs. They come not only to welcome your loved one, but to console you if you will let them. One of the frequent results of the death for caregivers is that a numbness takes over, protecting you from feeling the full impact of your grief. This effect is truly angelic, protecting you from further pain until you can handle it. Whether it stems from our own mind or from the intervention of spiritual beings, it can be a welcome relief. This is a time when imagination can be your friend. Whether you believe in angels or not, it is safe to go with your feelings at this time.

The varieties of spiritual belief are as diverse as the people subscribing to them. Most Americans, if polls are to be believed, not only believe in angels, but have had some communication during their lives with these beings. It does not really matter whether you believe in their actual existence or not, just as it doesn't matter whether they believe in your existence. The effects of their presence happen regardless of your belief. If you have no belief in angels, you can look at their presence simply as personifications of your own mental state and that of your loved one. As you give him up, it is helpful to assume that there will be one to receive him, as every gift implies both giver and recipient.

Finally there is you, and your loved one is gone, and the grief that wells up inside of you cannot be consoled. You may be numb for a time, but eventually your mind will allow you to experience your grief. You may be one who suffers in silence, privately, or you may be more demonstrative. Either way, your grief will seem as though it will never end.

Now is not the time to tell you that you will get better. Although grief does become less immediate, it does not ever fully go away. Your memories of your loved one will become treasures, because those feelings are a testament that you have lived and loved, a testament to the deep well of your humanity.

8 ◊◊ *Your Memorial or Funeral Service*

It is a far, far better thing that I do, than I have ever done;
it is a far, far better rest that I go to, than I have ever known.
CHARLES DICKENS, A TALE OF TWO CITIES

To the One Facing Death   ◊◊

Many people feel uncomfortable planning or contemplating their own funeral. At the same time, many feel anxiety at the thought that their funeral will not be the way they would like it to be. We normally think of the funeral as a service or program performed at the time of burial or cremation. A memorial service is more flexible as to time, since it can take place at any point after death and is sometimes many months or even years afterward. Many religious traditions have particular times when memorial services are deemed appropriate. Whichever you choose, you have a great many options.

To the Caregiver ✒

Like those facing death, caregivers often have difficulty with advance planning for the funeral or memorial service. It may seem disloyal to think about these things while your loved one is still alive. Even so, making plans for a funeral can be a time of bonding and an opportunity to clear up any misconceptions or misunderstandings between the two of you regarding this very important time. In Jewish tradition, accompanying someone to burial is one of the highest moral commandments. The sages say that it is truly a selfless act, because it cannot be repaid by the one who has died. The memorial service is the moment when the dying time ends and the period of mourning begins.

Funeral customs vary widely in our diverse population. The factors of cost, formality, and convenience are issues that will need to be addressed as you plan the service. We urge you to see to these arrangements before your loved one passes on, since the period surrounding the death will be one of great emotional turmoil. That is not the time to be making those decisions. The funeral is the last opportunity your loved one will have to make a statement about his life and his values, and it is important that his wishes be carried out.

The Obituary ✒

One of the first things that must be dealt with after your loved one has died is deciding whether there will be an announcement of the death in the local newspaper or other appropriate publication. It is a good idea to have the obituary written prior to death, so that you will not have to be creative at such an emotional time. Each publication has its own rules on what is customary and acceptable in death announcements. Some papers will not print the cause of death. Others will not include the names of survivors beyond the traditional family. If you know what is permitted, it will make composing the obituary easier and may avoid hurt feelings when the announcement appears. Many funeral homes take care of notifying the newspapers and utilize a fax for the purpose. If you have the obituary typed, or hand printed in large block letters, the staff at the paper will be able to avoid misspellings or misunderstandings.

We have included in the appendix several formats that you may find useful in preparing the obituary. Generally, the obituary includes the name of the deceased, possibly the cause of death, any relevant information about his education or work experience, and the survivors, including friends and caregivers. How many such names to include will, of course, depend on how long you want the obituary to be, and some publications charge either by the line or the word.

Planning the Service   ∞

While the funeral service may be largely dictated by custom if your loved one belongs to a religious tradition, there are a wide array of options concerning the format of the service, where his body is buried or the ashes scattered, and the basic formality of the event. If your loved one is not part of a formal religious community, the choices are even wider.

While it is true that the funeral service is a statement about the life and values of the person who has died, it is important to remember that the funeral is also for the living. It is a last good-bye from the deceased and also the beginning of mourning for the survivors. It should be an occasion of love, respect, and unity for all concerned. It should not be a time for getting even or for the living and their concerns to displace the memorial of the virtues of the deceased. The funeral is for the living, but it is *about* the one who died. We have seen funerals that made a mockery of the values of the one who died, and curiously, when that has happened, the living, too, have had a burden of dishonesty that they carry with them through their time of grief.

Your loved one may not wish to discuss his funeral arrangements. Planning a funeral, especially your own, is a direct contemplation of imminent death. Many find this difficult, whether the reluctance stems from a sense of denial or a fear of causing pain. Discussing these issues in a sensitive way, letting your loved one know that you are willing to talk about them when he is ready, takes courage but also will relieve everyone's mind about the arrangements. Your loved one may be willing to talk about his funeral months or weeks prior to his death, and he may never be able to talk about it. Often, clergy may provide the bridge for such a discussion. If possible, we encourage you as caregiver to participate in this discussion, so that you and the other survivors will know what is wanted.

We have heard and seen horror stories about the lover or special friends of the deceased being shut out of the funeral or memorial service. Even those who have been together in a relationship for many years have been treated with a cruelty beyond belief, and since they are not in the traditional relationship of spouse or close family, they have no legal rights whatever. It is for this reason that communication is essential, among all the parties, including the one who is dying. Fortunately there are some legal options that can deal with these matters.

We have spoken previously about the necessity of having a

durable power of attorney and a last will and testament. The one facing death has the right to designate in writing anyone he wishes to take care of his funeral arrangements and to decide what will be done and by whom. The person chosen need not be a relative. These provisions should be included in the last will and testament, since the authority granted under the durable power of attorney ceases at the time of death. If a provision granting custody of the body is not made, then the immediate family will have the legal right to decide what will be done. If your loved one is in any nontraditional family arrangement, then these matters should be taken care of before death occurs. This is especially true if it is known that there will be conflict among the survivors. Clear lines of authority may not completely remove the conflict, but at least everyone will know that what is done is being done according to the wishes of the deceased. Failing to make adequate provisions that will protect all of the survivors can cause a memorial service or funeral to be a time of anger and trouble, again putting the emotions and concerns of others ahead of those of the deceased. In death, as in life-facing-death, the dying person is at the center of the production.

In planning a memorial service, many factors must be considered. How long should it last? A funeral is a time of great emotion for most people. We think it appropriate, therefore, that the service be dignified but fairly brief, certainly lasting no more than an hour. Quite often the funeral will take place somewhere other than graveside, so transportation for the mourners becomes an added inconvenience and expense. Sometimes there will be no graveside service, or there will be one different from the funeral, such as military honors or a Masonic service. Some traditions tend to make the graveside service the principal one.

Another issue to face is the arrangement of donations or flowers. The lavish floral displays common to funerals several decades ago have become less popular, with the deceased and the survivors often preferring donations to some cause that the deceased has been involved in. However, flowers in our culture are a beautiful symbol of comfort and continuing life, so this is another area where there is no right answer. Frequently the obituary appearing in the paper will have the name and address of the charity your loved one has selected to receive memorial contributions. A charity usually acknowledges the gifts to the family of the deceased, so that the family may respond to those who have made donations. Arrangements can be made, though they are not necessary, with the selected charity prior to the death, so that it will know to expect the donations.

Music is important to most people, having as it does the ability to transcend space and time. For many, particular music or songs provide an instant connection to some past event or person. Why we like what we like in music is mysterious, an emotional connection beyond rational analysis. The music selected for a memorial service is therefore an important statement by the person who has died to those who have survived him. There can be no such thing as inappropriate music at a funeral. The music selected by your loved one, or his survivors, is making his statement, whatever that statement is. It is his statement and his alone.

∞ ∞ ∞ ∞ ∞ ∞ ∞ ∞ ∞ ∞ ∞ ∞ ∞ ∞ ∞ ∞ ∞

David: Denny was a good friend who told me months before his death that he wanted show tunes to be played at his funeral. As he was not in any way ill, I didn't pay much attention at the time. Little did we know that he had a serious heart condition, and just a short time later he had a massive heart attack and died.

When I arrived at the funeral home, I heard Broadway tunes playing over the sound system. What a wonderful tribute to this man! How fortunate that he had discussed his wishes with his wife, even though thoughts of death were far away. Of course, there were those who thought that kind of music was inappropriate, but it was what he wanted and beautifully summed up his carefree and happy approach to life.

∞ ∞ ∞ ∞ ∞ ∞ ∞ ∞ ∞ ∞ ∞ ∞ ∞ ∞ ∞ ∞ ∞ ∞

At the funeral, some people will feel comfortable only if they are dressed in formal clothes. It is still the custom in many places to wear black to a funeral, and wearing distinctive clothing can give you an instant and experiential connection to the deceased, as it can during an extended period of mourning.

You may choose duties to perform during the funeral, such as giving a eulogy. This should be a time for you to recall and celebrate the memory of your loved one and also to help others feel the depth of their loss. It is not inappropriate to include amusing stories as long as you bear in mind the feelings of other mourners. There is normally a period of time between the death and the funeral, and this time can be utilized not only to prepare what you wish to say, but to talk to others who want to give a eulogy. Stories told in this context can often acquire new importance and meaning and will be welcomed by the other mourners.

If you come from a religious background that is liturgical, then you might ask the clergy if you can participate in a formal way during the funeral. This can include reading Scripture, preparing a homily on the Scripture readings, participating in the distribution of communion, or ushering in the mourners. Most clergy will try their best to accommodate your wishes.

Religious and spiritual traditions have differing customs about what happens during the time surrounding the death and funeral. These customs can and should provide you a framework within which to express your grief. But no matter what the family traditions may be, you should be prepared to be shocked or hurt by things that people may say. Such comments are not usually meant to be hurtful, but they can be nonetheless.

In trying to comfort you, people sometimes say things like "Well, he's better off now" or "You'll get over it; try not to let it get you down." In reality, the people who say these things are trying to comfort themselves, not you. If they deny your pain and grief, then psychologically they believe this death won't cause them pain. Funerals are occasions when people say things they would never say in any other context. You may be a victim of this at your most vulnerable moment. Feel free to express the grief you feel, while trying to smooth over the rough spots as best as you can. This is now your time, a time of deep emotional suffering, and you are not required to look after the needs and feelings of anyone else. Let other people take care of you, not the other way around.

If you have a traditional way of expressing grief that is meaningful to you, then by all means go ahead with it. Some mourning customs have lapsed in our more informal society, but some of them can provide an emotional connection to the deceased and his memory.

Family and friends usually meet for a meal following the funeral. It is best if this can be arranged so that other people take care of the meal preparation and clean up afterward. This meal provides another opportunity to share stories about your loved one. For many, this meal will be the last event of the day, and everyone will be exhausted. Try not to schedule anything else until everyone has had a chance to rest and collect themselves.

Participation by the Deceased ⚭

Thanks to the miracles of modern communication, it has become possible for the deceased to take part in his own memorial service, through videotape, audiotape, or even photographs and slides. We have attended funerals where the deceased had made a videotape for his loved ones or had recorded the songs to be used at the funeral on audiotape. The use of videotape is increasingly common, since a visual image is much more powerful than just sound or a still photo. It truly seems to make the person who has died present for his loved ones.

⚭ ⚭ ⚭ ⚭ ⚭ ⚭ ⚭ ⚭ ⚭ ⚭ ⚭ ⚭ ⚭ ⚭ ⚭ ⚭ ⚭

Joan: Edward was a singer who had enjoyed a considerable amount of success in Nashville. He was aware that his life was drawing to a close as a result of heart disease. His music had shaped his life and career, and he enjoyed singing in his church choir. Long before his illness took its toll on his health and functioning, he persuaded his choir to sing backup for him in recording an old spiritual, "Ain't Got Time to Die." He quietly put aside the tape, and then, at his memorial service months later, we all had the glorious opportunity of hearing him sing one last time. I can't remember ever hearing a piece of music sung with so much feeling. The recording allowed Edward to sing at his own memorial, and he had asked a friend to provide copies of the recording for anyone who wanted one. I still enjoy my copy, and it is a beautiful remembrance and testimony to Edward and his enormous talent.

ﾞﾞﾞﾞﾞﾞﾞﾞﾞﾞﾞﾞﾞﾞﾞﾞﾞ

The use of video can be upsetting to survivors. If the one facing death wants to explore the use of video, it should be discussed with his loved ones. Seeing his image at the funeral and hearing his voice may be doubly traumatic for those who have just seen him through his illness and death. A great deal depends upon how familiar his loved ones may be with the uses of video. If he believes that a videotape may be too disturbing, it is possible to use slides taken throughout life, with accompanying music or commentary, either from him or his loved ones.

He may also choose to include a photo in the printed program for the service and a personal message to those who have gathered to attend his memorial. While this format will, of necessity, be brief, the inclusion of a personal message, or a poem or story meaningful to him, can be an effective way to communicate with those who have survived.

Options for Honoring the Body

We believe that the body is to be revered, that it is due the greatest honor and respect. While the ravages of disease or injury may have played havoc with its physical condition, it still is the ultimate expression of life, of matter infused with consciousness. Many people have definite ideas about what constitutes respect for the body. We have all heard people say, "Oh, I just couldn't be cremated" (or buried, or whatever taboo is being trod upon). Of course, the person who has died, at that point, probably doesn't care what is done to the body, but you can't know that. What we can know is what the deceased wanted before he died, and you can try to carry out those wishes.

Burial

In America today the custom of burial, going all the way back to prehistoric times, is still favored by a majority of people, though there are significant regional variations in burial practices. The East and West Coasts are more inclined to opt for cremation, while those living in the South and Midwest tend to opt for burial. Generally speaking, most Christian and all Jewish religious groups prefer burial. Many churches have been more accepting of cremation as time has gone on, but the symbolism of the eventual resurrection of the body is still powerful for many people. It was originally thought that cremation in some way denied the idea of resurrection, but that concern has faded over time. For Jews, the idea of cremation, after the Holocaust, has not been acceptable, plus there is a strong tradition of not destroying or desecrating the body, which cremation is felt to do.

The traditional funeral and burial have many advantages, from allowing a suitably dignified service to providing a place for the survivors to go during their period of mourning. Psychologically it can be useful for the mourners to accompany the body to burial. It makes the loss all the more stark and therefore real. In a very physical way, the person who has died is present for the mourners, and this can be beneficial to them as they adjust to the loss.

Many decisions will need to be made about the funeral, and the person who is facing death should participate in those decisions as much as he is able and willing. Seemingly mundane concerns such as the clothes to be worn can figure prominently in the mind of your loved one. Where the burial should take place is another matter that is frequently important to the dying. Many families assume they know what their loved one would want regarding his funeral and frequently are surprised to learn that they are wrong. It is best to talk things through.

While the traditional funeral and burial have many advantages, there are drawbacks. Chief among these is the expense. Everything about the traditional funeral can be costly. There is the cost of the casket, rental for the funeral home, transportation to the cemetery, and the burial itself. There is also the purchase of the plot and frequently a onetime charge for the future maintenance of the gravesite. As in any business transaction, get all costs in writing to avoid misunderstandings and trouble later.

CREMATION

Cremating the body has become an increasingly favored option in the United States. It has the advantage of being less costly than a traditional funeral and burial. Usually funeral homes will arrange for cremation for a set fee, and in many places the survivors may be present at the cremation if they wish to do so. In some places a casket is still required, but obviously the least expensive one is appropriate in such a case. In most cases, no casket is required. Additionally, no plot is necessary, with its attendant expense and upkeep. A variety of urns to hold the ashes is available, either from the funeral home or purchased separately. Some people keep the ashes, or a portion of them, for a long time, while others prefer to dispose of them shortly after the memorial service. There is no right way or wrong way to take care of these matters.

Many people like to have a place where they can go to recall the one who has died. Cremation does not take away this opportunity. Wherever the ashes are, then that place will forever be associated with the deceased in the minds of his survivors. In some way, the place where the remains of our loved ones rest is a place where we can commune with their spirits and recall our memories of them.

In terms of organizing a memorial service around a cremation, the issues are virtually the same as for the more traditional funeral. The only thing that will be absent, normally, is the body, though it can be arranged for the body to be cremated after the service rather than before. If the body has already been cremated, then often the ashes, accompanied perhaps by a picture of your loved one, will be present at the service.

When and how—or whether—to dispose of the ashes of your loved one is really up to you. You may wish to be alone at this time, or you may want other friends or family to be present. We know of one instance where the friends of the dead man took small portions of his ashes all over the world and disposed of them in his favorite places. There is no requirement that the ashes (or cremains) be disposed of in any particular manner, time, or place. Some choose to have their ashes scattered over the ocean, over a favorite river or lake, or in some peaceful, quiet place. The whereabouts should be decided, if possible, in consultation with your loved one, if he has any wishes in this regard at all. On the other hand, this particular issue will have more impact on the survivors than on the one who is dying. It is they who must see themselves through their grief, and if they have strong feelings about what should be done with the ashes, then those feelings should probably carry considerable weight unless their loved one has indicated otherwise.

Whatever your choices are, we hope that you will use the funeral or memorial service to deepen your spiritual connection to your loved one. Your relationship to your loved one does not cease when he dies, but it changes. You will not see one another again in the flesh, but your relationship will not cease to exist just because one of you has died. Even if you do not believe in a world-to-come, your loved one will live on in your memory.

9 ✿ Counting on Life to Heal the Grief

you left
traces
of your self
all over my room:
a poem scribbled in the
margin of a book
a corner of a page
turned over in another book.
where are you tonight?
in whose room are you leaving
traces?
are you perhaps
discovering
the traces of my self I left on your soul?

PETER McWILLIAMS

To the One Facing Death ✿

This chapter is written primarily for your caregivers and family who have surrounded you. While we hope to help you and them find meaning and dignity through this time of crisis, nothing will mitigate their feelings of loss and despair. Like all plays, this one will have its final act and curtain. There is nothing you can do to lessen their pain, and you are not responsible for doing so. In a way, their grief at your going is a living testament to the value of your life and your love. You will be missed, and you will be remembered.

To the Caregiver

There are many levels of grief, from the profound emptiness of losing a spouse or a child, to the expected but irreplaceable loss of a parent, to the loss of friends. You alone know the depth of your grief, for grief, like pain, is an intensely private affair. The end of the dying time is the beginning of mourning, and mourning, for those in profound grief, is a full-time job. For those having less emotional attachment to the dying person, the process of grief and loss may be less devastating but is nevertheless acute and real.

The Stages of Grief

Just as there are emotional states you pass through in the course of dying, so there are stages of grief within the time of mourning. While we discuss these, bear in mind that you cannot expect to have them in the nice, neat order described. You may be in several stages at once, and some you may never realize you have at all. Mourning is a process that is unique to every individual. The feelings you have at this time are honest; they will not betray you. Your task at this time is to care for those feelings. No one ever had a dishonest emotion at a time such as this.

For weeks or months, you have faced the impending loss of your loved one, and now that day has arrived. The phrase "anticipatory grieving" has been used in previous chapters, and undoubtedly you have had some of those feelings of panic, anger, isolation, and guilt. Even though we use the word "grieving" to summarize those feelings, the emotional state following a death is quite different. Many of those feelings will no longer be there. Even if we believe we are prepared, there is a part of us that shouts a great, cosmic "No!" at the death of our loved one.

DENIAL

And so, the first stage of mourning is denial. You have known, intellectually, that your loved one was dying. You have known this since you were first told of his diagnosis. You have cared for him over the weeks and months. You have cried; you have hurled your defiance at the universe. You have held his hand while he was dying. And you watched as his life force ebbed away, as his spirit was liberated from his suffering body. What room is there for denial?

There is room for denial because we do not always internalize what we know. Even when we behold the lifeless body of our loved one, somehow we cannot take it in. One of the thoughtless things someone may say to you is, "It's not the end of the world." But it is, in fact, the end of the world you have known.

Three things that cause life-threatening stress are the loss of a job, divorce, and the death of a loved one. The loss of a job threatens our self-esteem. A divorce destroys a relationship that was, at one time, the center of our lives. The death of a loved one can be even more profound.

In every relationship there is a "you," a "me," and an "us." In divorce, the "us" is destroyed, while "you" and "me" go on. When a loved one dies, not only is the "us" destroyed, but the "you" is gone also. If it is your spouse who dies, the center of your life is ripped away, leaving you with nothing more than shreds of memory.

The mystery here is not that we react with denial, but that

we can survive at all. It is precisely the denial that enables us to live through the first onslaught of grief.

It is not unusual for the mind to block out all thoughts of the deceased during the initial stages of mourning. You know what has occurred, but you can't focus your mind on the actual death and the trauma leading up to it. The mind can't stand that much pain at once, and only slowly, over time, will it permit you to experience the depth of your loss.

ISOLATION

Another stage, commonly occurring throughout the first stages of mourning, is isolation. You are sure that nobody has ever felt this bad before, that nobody can understand what you are going through. In a certain sense, no one can.

You are unique, as your loved one was unique. The "us" of your relationship was unique, made up of all of your hopes, your fears, your love, and your experiences. This is true whether your loved one was your lover, your child, or your friend. No one ever had that relationship before, and no one ever will again. The grief that you now feel, in a very real sense, has never been felt by anyone else. No one else *can* understand.

Thus this isolation, from one perspective, is frightening. How can we be helped if no one knows where we are? And this isn't a situation where nobody *does* know, but one where they *cannot* know. You are alone.

There is, however, another perspective. You aren't really alone, because your loved one is there with you. Your grief is your last experience of your loved one, the last thing you share. In a very real sense, it is your connection to him. Therefore this isolation is something to be not feared, but embraced. The depth of your grief is your testimony to the strength of your love. Do not flee from it! Do not let others minimize what you are feeling. Your grief is yours, not theirs.

Think of all the relationships your loved one had. Perhaps you were his spouse, his confidant, his lover. Your grief will be different from that suffered by his mother, his son, his business associate, his best friend. Each one of you experienced him differently, so now your grieving will be different. For some, the difference will be not only in degree, but in kind. The relationships of parents to children are special ones. The life sharing that takes place between life partners or spouses is the very deepest that can occur. The special bond of friendship that may have existed between your loved one and his best, his closest friend can't be understood by anyone else.

The way you experience your loss will also be different from that of other people. What will work for some will not work for others. In a very real way you *are* isolated, and you have to find your own way out, but others may be able to help. A shoulder to cry on, a kind word or deed, may make the pain more bearable, but no one can show you the way to go.

This is not to minimize the isolation that can be imposed from the outside, from your circle of friends and family. Even people who share your grief may exclude you without really meaning to. Many find it difficult to talk about a loved one who has died, and if you mention your grief or the one who has died, they may change the subject or minimize your grief.

Refusal to talk about the deceased, or even mention his name, is like shutting a steel door on the grief-stricken. They have no way of working through the grief they feel. Like stuffed anger, stuffed grief has to come out in some way, frequently through causing illness. Regardless of how momentarily embarrassing talk about your loved one may be, it is a lot easier than dealing with serious health problems later.

❁ ❁ ❁ ❁ ❁ ❁ ❁ ❁ ❁ ❁ ❁ ❁ ❁ ❁ ❁ ❁ ❁ ❁ ❁

David: After my friend Lynn died, I remained close to his mother. We had struggled together to care for Lynn during his illness. The night he died, his mother and I stood the death watch together. She told me, "We started this together, and we need to finish this together."

I have been able to go visit with her at least a couple of times every year, and I always call her on December 20, the day Lynn died.

On one trip she said to me, "I'm so glad when you come up to see me. No one here will talk to me about Lynn."

What a sad commentary, but I found that it is typical in that region of the country. "Your loved one is dead, he's buried, you have to get on with your life." That is just not the way I experience grief. I need to talk about it, I need to work through my grief, and that takes time.

❁ ❁ ❁ ❁ ❁ ❁ ❁ ❁ ❁ ❁ ❁ ❁ ❁ ❁ ❁ ❁ ❁ ❁ ❁

ANGER

For many of us, anger is a difficult emotion. Society often disapproves of anger, and some of us have spent our lives dealing with it. We hide or block the anger we feel, and after a lifetime we may believe that we no longer feel it. When a loved one dies, our emotions can boil over in an uncontrollable rush. We are so vulnerable, in such pain, that we may believe we, too, are dying.

It is all right to feel anger at this time. You may be angry at your loved one for leaving you, perhaps for not caring for himself in a way that would have prolonged his life. You may be angry at God or Goddess, the fates, or society. You may be angry at the doctors for not being able to prevent his death. All of these feelings are normal and human.

Many people are appalled at the notion that they could be angry with God. Some have lost their faith at the death of a loved one, unable to believe in a Being who could allow such a loss and such grief. All the human beings who have ever lived had times when they were angry with God. Anger is a healthy emotion, and denying anger creates stress, and stress causes negative health consequences, not at all what a loving Creator would want. If you feel somehow that God has not lived up to his part of the bargain, not fulfilled the terms of his covenant with you, then you will feel angry. He is an adult, He can take it. The heavens will not shake, lightning will not flash. Just as you can be angry with your parent, sibling, or lover, and still love them, so you can be angry at God and still love him.

The question is, what can you do with your anger? It may be not the garden-variety, you-left-your-wet-towel-on-the-bathroom-floor-type anger, but a cosmic rage that may manifest itself in all kinds of unpleasant ways.

ıɔɔ ıɔɔ ıɔɔ ıɔɔ ıɔɔ ıɔɔ ıɔɔ ıɔɔ ıɔɔ ıɔɔ ıɔɔ ıɔɔ ıɔɔ ıɔɔ ıɔɔ ıɔɔ ıɔɔ ıɔɔ

David: Over the course of ten and more years of caregiving, I have come to know many people at the most intimate moments of their lives. The cumulative losses have generated in me waves of grief and despair and not a little anger. I have been fortunate in having friends and family who have allowed me to talk about what I have felt and to express my grief. I felt that I was handling these tides of emotion pretty well.

A year ago I woke up one morning, and the first thought in my mind was, I'm so tired of being angry! I realized how bitter I had become, both at the fact of my losses and because I was still alive myself. Realizing that the source of the anger was the grief I felt, I could let it go. Anger is an exhausting emotion, one that is usually not socially acceptable and one we tend to suppress. I have found that therapy with a good social worker, talking with understanding friends, and meditation have enabled me to work through my feelings of anger and despair and to pick up and return to the battle.

ᔈᖉ ᔈᖉ ᔈᖉ ᔈᖉ ᔈᖉ ᔈᖉ ᔈᖉ ᔈᖉ ᔈᖉ ᔈᖉ ᔈᖉ ᔈᖉ ᔈᖉ ᔈᖉ ᔈᖉ ᔈᖉ ᔈᖉ ᔈᖉ

Recognizing that you have the anger is one thing, but deciding what to do with it is another. Writing about your anger can be psychologically beneficial. You may express your feelings completely and honestly on paper, without offending anyone. If you want, tear up the paper after you have finished. Actually, tearing up what you have written may help you to let go of the anger you feel.

Other options include talking with your friends about how you feel, if they will let you. You may go to a quiet place and scream or cry or beat pillows with your fists. The only rule is, you may not cause injury to yourself or any other living thing. Actually, breaking something—something you don't need—can help allow you to release your anger. The important thing is to find a way to express the anger you feel and to let go of it. It will make you sick if you don't.

DEPRESSION

The tremendous flood of emotions that you are experiencing will inevitably lead to feelings of depression. There is nothing wrong with this as long as you avoid the clinical state of depression and eventually transform the depression into acceptance and hope.

We need to be clear that the feeling of being depressed, of being sad, is not the same thing as the more serious illness called major depression. The former is probably inevitable; the latter is not. Clinical depression is characterized by a general listlessness, a lack of interest in your life or energy to do anything, difficulty sleeping (or sleeping too much), and trouble with addictive substances such as alcohol, tobacco, drugs, or food. It may be accompanied by thoughts of suicide or a wish to do harm to others, and it may require professional intervention.

You may have never been as sad as you are right now. Depending on the level of emotional involvement you had with your loved one, this feeling may go on for a very long time. It would not be unusual for you to have some of the symptoms of clinical depression such as a loss of interest in the thousands of details of everyday living that normally fill our lives. You may be uninterested in watching the television or reading the newspaper. You may have little appetite. You may find it difficult to concentrate, and your memory may be impaired temporarily. You may find that you want to speak to some of your friends, but not others. In short, instead of the nice, neat little package that your life usually resembles, it may feel erratic and disordered. This is normal, and you need not be afraid of it. You have just gone through an emotional ordeal, and it will take time—often a good deal of it—for you to put your life back together. As you work through your grief, pay attention to your emotional state and to that of the other mourners around you. No one ever said this would be easy, and you or others may need help in dealing with it. If you are showing symptoms of more serious depression that is not getting better during the year after the death, or if you are contemplating suicide, you may have left a state of healthy grieving and become seriously clinically depressed. If this happens, get help immediately.

In the midst of your sadness, remember that your loved one would not wish you to suffer more. The pain of separation is inevitable, and that pain will cause you sadness, but you are still alive and you must go on living. Many hospices and hospitals have grief support groups to help the bereaved work through the sadness.

The hole in your heart caused by this loss may never be filled. You may not want it to be filled. For many, the loss of a spouse or a child may be inconsolable. But you can learn to live with the loss. And just as you can learn to live with physical pain, you can learn to live with emotional pain. Nobody likes it, and *you* don't have to like it, but you have an obligation to yourself, to your loved one, and to those still living around you to reenter the land of the living, after your time of grief.

ACCEPTANCE AND HOPE

As we have said, the depth of your grief will have a direct relationship to your emotional attachment to your loved one. Medical personnel, even while trying to maintain professional objectivity, may still (and often do) form an emotional bond with the dying. You may have been intimately involved in the care of your loved one, or you may have been a supportive outsider, involved only tangentially in his care. Whatever your place in the grand scheme of things, and the degree of your mourning, it will eventually resolve into acceptance and hope.

Many books dealing with grieving speak of recovery. We

have deliberately avoided using this term, since recovery implies a return to a healthy state. Mourning is not an unhealthy state; in fact, it is unavoidable. Nor will you return to a state of health resembling what you had before your loved one died. Your life is forever altered by his death—not altogether in a bad way. In fact, your new perspectives on life may make it more real, more honest. But it will never be the same again.

How long does it take to reach the stage of acceptance? That cannot be predicted. It depends on the depth of your emotional attachment to the one who has died and on your own emotional state. Your physical and mental health may be factors as well as the outlets you have to express your grief.

Thus, mourning may last for months or it may continue for years. For some, it will last for the remainder of their lives. However, it does become less immediate, less dominating in our lives.

In the period immediately following death, when numbness takes over, you will not experience the full impact of your loss. That may come days or weeks later, as your mind allows you to understand what has happened. The feeling of being terribly sad and depressed may not come for months. Your anger may be felt for an extended period of time.

You will realize that you are reaching the stage of acceptance when you begin to take an interest in life again. When this happens, it may be accompanied by a feeling of betrayal as you move further away from your loved one. You may try to recall your feelings of grief, but over time they will fade and you will be able to think about other things. Gradually you will begin making plans again.

Acceptance does not imply forgetting your loved one or the relationship you shared. It is the slow but sure recognition that you are still alive and that you can go on living. It is a gradual cessation of your constant inward-directed thoughts and an ability to focus on things outside of yourself.

With acceptance comes hope. Why hope? Because when we are in the depths of grief, we can give in to despair, the feeling that we are never going to feel good again. That feeling will pass. With its passing, hope will return.

What can you hope for? That depends upon where you are. If you are elderly, you may hope for a bright, happy future for your children and grandchildren. You may hope for another relationship, not a replacement for what you've lost, but a new adventure altogether. If you have lost a child, you may hope for a brighter future for your other children or, if you are young enough, perhaps for another child. If you have lost a parent, you may hope to see his ideals manifested in your own life and that of your children.

In the Greek myth, when Pandora opened the box, all the horrible goblins of misery and starvation, death, destruction, and disease flew out and filled the world. In despair, Pandora sat on the box and wept. Then she heard a gentle tapping from inside the box. She feared to open the box again, given what had just happened, but her curiosity got the better of her, and she lifted the lid just a little. Inside she saw a little white dove, emblematic of hope. Hope is gentle, hope is unobtrusive, hope is what is left over after all the bad things that you experience in this life. Hope is a consolation in the present and a promise for the future. You will find hope again.

Multiple Losses ✎

While a death may be a profound individual tragedy, most people have to deal with death only on an infrequent basis.

There are those, however, who deal with loss as a regular part of their lives. They have special concerns in dealing with grief.

The elderly have long known that the years late in life are filled with loss. As a ninety-year-old friend said, "If you live long enough, and you don't make younger friends, you'll be the last one left that you know." Another said, "I know more dead people than living ones." Chronic grief and loss are the principal reasons for depression among the elderly. They often have feelings of loss of hope for a future and waiting in line to see who will be next to die.

These feelings are not unique to the elderly. Others deeply affected by multiple losses, but seldom acknowledged as experiencing that pain, are nurses, physicians, social workers, ministers and other helping professionals, and even nonprofessional caregivers who work with the dying.

Physicians are particularly affected, because they are trained to try to prevent death, so in addition to all of the painful emotions of other caregivers, they also experience feelings of failure and inadequacy when a patient dies.

Nurses generally spend more time with the dying than other health care providers. Nurses are more likely to be comfortable when a patient is ready to die, because they know that their nursing care is just as important at that point. Although nurses are much less likely to see death as a failure on their part, they frequently experience the loss personally. Many nurses burn out after only a few years in practice because of the cumulative effect of multiple losses.

Caregivers who are able to continue working with the dying find their own methods for surviving. Hospice caregivers experience a low rate of burnout and staff turnover. They are known to be generally cheerful, happy people. Their secret is that they have confronted their own mortality and are comfortable with death and the meaning it has for them as individuals.

Other ways to avoid burnout are to set realistic goals and to express thoughts and feelings about each death as it occurs. If your goal is to save the person with a terminal illness, you will fail every time. Your job isn't to save, but to care for and love. You can always succeed in these things. When you talk about the experiences you had with the deceased, and express your feelings of loss, you will feel better, more alive, and more whole for having done so. In the end, you will be able to look back and remember the joy, the intimacy, the privilege it was to be able to help, to love, and to care. And you will be able to continue to provide care to others.

⋈ ⋈ ⋈ ⋈ ⋈ ⋈ ⋈ ⋈ ⋈ ⋈ ⋈ ⋈ ⋈ ⋈ ⋈ ⋈ ⋈ ⋈

Joan: "An angel from Angela to an Angel," said the card, decorated with one of Raphael's angels, coming just two months before Angela's death several years ago. And it finally hit me. I *can* actually do something with the accumulated grief of losing a thousand patients/clients through my years in nursing. And the Angel Project was born.

The chronic loss of patients can have devastating consequences on us as health care professionals. All of the techniques that had worked for me through the years were beginning to wear thin when Angela sent me my angel card. She had particularly liked the logo for my practice, a butterfly emerging from the chrysalis. I decided with Angela's inspiration to begin the Angel Project. The Angel Project is a journal (that happens to have Raphael's angel on the front) in which I memorialize each patient who dies. I write an entry when I am ready for closure. This could be within hours or days after the death, or later, depending on the nature of the relationship. I write each entry as a letter to the patient. I include things I particularly liked about her, and I thank her for the lessons she taught me or the privilege of having her in my life. Any unsaid words or regrets are included as well. Any mementos are enclosed, such as pictures, notes, or cards, programs from performances, or obituaries. All the remaining evidence in my personal possession about this person goes in the Angel Project.

The Angel Project provides closure, without which I would repeat an old mistake. Twenty years after Vietnam, standing at the memorial, I could only recall the name of one of dozens of friends lost there. Human life is too precious to be forgotten, even for those of us who are midwives of the exit.

࿒ ࿒ ࿒ ࿒ ࿒ ࿒ ࿒ ࿒ ࿒ ࿒ ࿒ ࿒ ࿒ ࿒ ࿒ ࿒ ࿒

Keeping Anniversaries ࿒

In many spiritual traditions it is customary to celebrate anniversaries, to keep the remembrance of the deceased alive. Judaism provides four opportunities each year to recall loved ones, and the bereaved recite certain blessings on the anniversary of the death. Christianity, too, provides for anniversaries of remembrance, most notably on All Souls Day, November 2. In Mexico and other Latin American cultures it is known as the Day of the Dead and is marked by widespread memorials to those who have died. Whatever your spiritual practice, you will find that fixed times for the remembrance of your loved one can be beneficial and can speed the process of acceptance.

Regardless of the formal requirements of the anniversary that your tradition may impose, this is a time to remember. If your loved one died near a particular holiday or family celebration, then those occasions may be associated forever in your memory.

What do we do on these anniversaries? Obviously the closer you are in time to the actual death, the more emotionally stressful these occasions will be. Even if the date slips your mind, your subconscious mind remembers, and you may experience increased dreams or unexpected or unexplained feelings of sadness or agitation on that date.

After the first flood of grief has passed, anniversaries are occasions that you can use to express your continued mourning. Most people will understand that you need to express this grief, and anniversaries are socially appropriate occasions to do this. You may gather your loved one's friends and family around you on these occasions and have the wonderful experience of transforming the pain of grief into the pleasure of memory. Allow yourself to feel and recall the good things as well as the bad.

Keepsakes and Remembrances 🕉

Mementos of your loved one will be treasured by all who cared about him, and he may in fact give away some of his personal belongings before his death to those he loves.

It is customary in many cultures to keep a lock of the deceased's hair, as the only physical part of him that it is acceptable to retain. When there has been a cremation, close family members or friends may want to keep a small portion of the ashes. Certainly we all have small objects or things that have great meaning for us, and family and friends may wish to share these.

Unfortunately the time for giving these items can be an occasion of conflict. Some people may want the same thing, or the surviving spouse or family may not want to part with some items. If this responsibility falls to you, then know that when and how personal items are distributed is solely up to you. You don't have to apologize if you aren't ready to deal with this topic at the time. Nor do you have to give away an item that may be loaded with memories for you just because somebody else wants it. The act of giving remembrances to people is an act of grace, to be performed as and when you are able.

You may find that being surrounded by your loved one's things is comforting, and you may hesitate to give them up. That is perfectly understandable. The things he valued, the clothes he wore, the toys he played with, are all a part of him and a part of you. Remember that even though you are immersed in your grief, other people will be mourning as well. It is a kindness to give others mementos of their particular relationship with your loved one, and it is something that he would have wanted.

Guarding Your Grief

Finally, you must learn to guard your grief. There will be those who will try to minimize your grief, to cheer you up when you don't want this to happen. This is an attempt at self-protection on their part, subconsciously assuming that if they minimize your grief, they will not feel their own sadness. This is not an intentional cruelty, but it can feel that way, particularly if it is carried on for a long period of time. Your grief is yours, and you have a right to have it.

As your grief begins to ease, you will need to guard it from yourself. By this, we mean that even though you will have to live with your mourning for a while, it is not meant to be a permanent living arrangement. It must be placed in perspective. You do not have to recall the pain every waking hour of every day, and over time you will see your emotional pain as just a part—an important part—of your life.

Grief is now an integral part of your loved one. Since it is the last thing that you shared, in a way, it is a most precious gift. It has often been noted that survivors tend in some way to deify their lost loved one. He will never make any mistakes again in this world, and you may tend to forget any negative qualities he may have had. The end of the mourning process may produce a memory that may have only a slight resemblance to the actual person who died. That is perfectly all right. You have the right to remember your loved one as you want to remember him. With or without warts, they are *your* memories, no one else's.

I shall miss loving you.
I shall miss the Comfort of your embrace.
I shall miss the
Loneliness of waiting for the
calls that never came.
I shall miss the Joy of your comings,
and the Pain of your goings
and,
after a time,
I shall miss
missing
loving
you.

PETER McWILLIAMS

10   *Closing the Circle*

That time of year thou mayst in me behold
When yellow leaves, or none, or few, do hang
Upon those boughs which shake against the cold,
Bare ruined choirs, where late the sweet birds sang.
In me thou see'st the twilight of such day
As after sunset fadeth in the west;
Which by and by black night doth take away,
Death's second self, that seals up all in rest.
In me thou see'st the glowing of such fire
That on the ashes of his youth doth lie,
As the death-bed whereon it must expire,
Consumed with that which it was nourish'd by.
   This thou perceivest, which makes thy love more strong,
   To love that well which thou must leave ere long.

WILLIAM SHAKESPEARE, SONNET LXXIII

The circle of life is eternal. It begins where it ends and ends where it begins; birthing and birth, growing and life, dying and death, birthing into new expanded awareness, new lives replacing those departed. Every day, in all life forms, as one leaves, another is born; as one phase of life passes, life surpasses itself. Death closes and thus completes the raw beauty of the circle as we are capable of seeing it while we are still alive.

However, in the midst of the tragedy of losing your own life or the life of one you love, it may be hard to conceive of a circle, or anything continuing or continuous. Your loss is too close, too tragic, perhaps, even to comprehend the circle of life. It may simply feel like a horrible and useless tragedy, or you may consider it as tragedy in the epic sense.

The word "tragedy" conjures images and feelings for all of us. If we look at Shakespeare, we see parallels to the real-life drama of the dying time. In these epic tragedies, there are three consistent characteristics. First are the noble characters whose lives cause them to be raised above the common concerns and normal life. In facing your death or in being a caregiver, you encounter and handle challenges far beyond what you believe yourself capable of, far beyond common concerns. Second, there is a tragic flaw that overcomes the hero and kills him; the hero always dies. For you this manifests as a flaw not of character, but of the physical body, causing imminent death. This physical flaw that cannot be overcome must be faced and accepted, and ultimately all must surrender to it.

The third characteristic of tragedy is the catharsis that arises from the realization that the world is a better place for the hero having been here. The way in which you face death leaves your special mark on the world. It empowers others to learn and grow. It engenders closeness and intimacy within the circle of family, friends, and supporters by allowing them to participate in the dying. The caregiver, too, helps a loved one who is dying in many ways that make her world better by allowing her to be in charge of her living and dying.

Each divine creation is both noble and beautiful and therefore the subject of tragedy when life is lost. In true tragedy, everyone experiences the full range of genuine caring to allevi-

ate suffering and expresses a life-changing emotional commit-
ment to the one who is dying.

We would like to close the circle with the words of Goethe:
"Every moment Nature starts on the longest journey, and every
moment she reaches her goal." The dying time is a time of living and learning and reaching for new goals. As you choreo-
graph your final act or help the one you love, who is dying, we
hope that you hold on to the light that you experience and that
you emerge as the life that surpasses itself.

∽ *Appendix*

Guided Imagery Scripts ∽

You may use these scripts to create a safe place in your mind. You may try this on your own or ask for help from a therapist, caregiver, or friend. Either way, we suggest that:

1. You read through the script and decide if it sounds okay to you.
2. Either ask someone to read the script to you each time or you or she may make a recording of the script. (It is much easier to relax if you are listening to your own voice or someone else's rather than trying to remember what to do next.)

3. As you record, remember to *slow down* and lower your natural speaking voice. Pause at the end of each phrase and sentence. Leave longer pauses where you are imagining doing something, such as standing under a waterfall. Talk in as soothing a voice as you can, as though you were speaking to a little child. If you want background music, choose something that won't change the beat, tempo, or pitch. Be sure that the music doesn't stop in the middle of the recording.

4. Turn off the phone and be sure that you have a safe and quiet place to record; it will take twenty minutes or so to read or record the imagery.

5. After you have recorded the imagery, practice the visualization several times, until the pattern becomes clear in your mind and your body responds automatically. If, at any time while listening, you feel uncomfortable, open your eyes and stop the imagery.

IMAGERY FOR CREATING A SAFE PLACE

Allow yourself to be in a comfortable position, either lying down or sitting up. Make sure that your body is well supported. Begin by taking a couple of long, deep breaths all the way down into your diaphragm. (Inhale.) Hold it, and as you exhale, let go of the tension. (Exhale.) Letting go. . . . Take another deep breath all the way in. (Inhale.) Allow all the tension to move into your lungs, and then let it go (exhale), just begin to let go. . . . And if you're still feeling tense, repeat this process a few times as you begin to let go, begin to relax. . . . Create a silent and healing space around you. . . . Focus only on your quiet breathing and the sound of my voice. . . . Allow yourself to begin to let go, to create a healing time, a time of peace and safety. . . .

I'm going to count from seven to one. And as I count, you'll find yourself becoming more and more relaxed. Relax your body . . . relax your mind . . . focus only on your breathing and the sound of my voice . . . and letting go. Seven. . . .

Relax your feet and ankles. Allow your feet and ankles to become very relaxed. Wiggle your toes to let the tension out. . . . Allow this relaxation to drift up into your calves and your knees, relaxing those muscles in your legs, even relaxing the bones. . . . Allow the relaxation to drift up into your thighs, relaxing those muscles in your thighs. And gently relax your hips and your pelvic area. Relax your lower abdomen all the way to your navel. . . . Relax your lower back. . . . Six. . . .

Let the relaxation gently drift. Let it drift up into your solar plexus area . . . and into your chest and your lungs, just letting go. . . . Let the relaxation surround your heart and your lungs, and relax. . . . Notice how gentle and quiet your breathing is becoming. . . . Let the relaxation drift around to your back. Relax each bone in your back, and all the muscles and all the nerves, as the relaxation fills your shoulders now, gently spilling over your shoulders and down to your elbows. . . . Relax your forearms and your wrists. . . . Relax the palms of your hands and your fingers. Five. . . .

Relax your neck . . . all that tension that holds your shoulders up, tight, around your ears. Let your shoulders drop now, and let the tension go. . . . Allow the relaxation to drift up the back of your scalp and into your head. . . . Each breath allows you to become more and more relaxed. Let the relaxation drift into your eyes, and your nose, and your cheeks. . . . Your mouth becomes so relaxed . . . your tongue relaxes enough to drop away from the roof of your mouth. Your jaw drops just a little. . . . You're so relaxed. And going deeper, you relax. Four. . . . Three. . . .

More and more relaxed. . . . And two. . . . Scan your body for any remaining pockets of tension. And let go. . . . And one. . . .

You find yourself in a safe place outdoors. Perhaps it's not a place you've ever seen before except in the beauty of your own mind. You see a place outdoors that is beautifully safe. . . . Allow the images to come. . . . For in this place of safety, only you are allowed. . . . In this place of safety, no one can come without your invitation. . . . In this place of safety, you are always at peace. . . .

Allow the images to come. . . . Notice the color of the sky at your favorite time of day. . . . And in this place, at this most perfect time of day, at the season and the temperature that you like on your skin . . . allow your senses to become more and more alive. Look around at the surroundings and allow yourself to see; if not with your eyes, then sense with your heart. . . . Each time you come to your safe place, you may develop it and allow it to become more and more beautiful. Allow yourself to see what is here today. . . . Notice the color of the trees or flowers or grass, or perhaps sand or water. Let the colors and textures come alive for you in this beautiful and safe place. . . .

Listen to the sounds of safety. . . . Perhaps you hear birds or splashing . . . or the sound of wind in the trees or the grass. . . . Allow yourself to create a place of safety and peace that is always yours, always safe. . . . And breathe in the safety. . . . And breathe out the fear. . . . And breathe in the safety. . . . And breathe out the fear. . . .

As you breathe in, you can even smell the smells of safety . . . perhaps salty air, or the sweet smell of a flower. . . . Breathe in the smells of your safe place. It's so safe here that you can even taste it as you lick your lips. Let yourself bask in the safety and the peace. . . .

Allow yourself to walk around . . . to be in this place . . . to notice more and more, to create more and more in this place. . . . Perhaps you would like to build a shelter of some kind, a cottage, a cave, a tent, a treehouse. And if it's already there, you may add to it. . . . Plant flowers, adding a splash of color. . . . Add special places or rooms to your safe place. . . . Create anything that you would like. (Long pause.)

Create special places for special kinds of feelings that need to be healed, special places to wash away fear and pain. . . . Create a waterfall or a pool of healing water. Stand under the waterfall to wash away the fear. . . . Let the healing waters wash away what you'd like to be finished with. Each time you come to the waterfall or the healing pool of water, you can wash away more and more of the past. . . . Each time you come, you are cleansed and rejuvenated . . . the fear and the pain are washed away. . . . Wash away the fear and pain. . . . Wash all of it away, as you are ready. (Long pause.) When you are finished, step out of the water and you will find a robe or a towel to dry and warm yourself. . . .

Now allow yourself to continue walking around your safe place. . . . You find a healing garden, a place that is just for healing your mind and spirit. . . . Here you can plant anything you would like. . . . You can plant wishes and dreams for your peace and safety. . . . You can plant seeds of healing your mind and spirit. And you can weed out what you want to be finished with. Take some time to work with your garden now. (Long pause.)

And now, find your favorite place in all of safety. Walk around until you find just the right place. (Long pause.) Sit down, and get comfortable. . . . Slowly breathe in the safety and the peace. Breathe out the fear. . . . Breathe in the safety and peace. Breathe out the fear. . . . Breathe in the safety and peace. . . . Breathe out the fear. . . . And just be in this place as you slowly breathe and heal your mind and spirit. . . .

Stay in this place as long as you would like. . . . And when you are ready, simply count yourself out by counting from one to five. When you reach the number five, your eyes will open. And you will be awake and alert and feeling safe and at peace.

Short Version of Imagery for Creating a Safe Place

(To the caregiver: This version or parts of it may be read or recited to your loved one, who is familiar with the previous longer version. It is useful in times of crisis or fear, when concentration is short term and you want to reduce fear quickly. It is helpful to read in a rhythm of her quiet breathing.)

Begin to breathe in the safety and peace. . . . Breathe out the fear. . . . And breathe in the safety and peace. . . . And breathe out the fear. . . . Each time you breathe in, relax your body. . . . And each time you exhale, let go of tension. . . . Breathe in relaxation. . . . Breathe out tension. . . . With each breath, begin to count. Make each breath a number. Five . . . four . . . three . . . two . . . one . . . each exhale letting go. As you are counting, as you are breathing, allow the image of safety to fill your mind. . . . You are there, in safety . . . in peace. . . . No one can be there with you without your permission. Focus only on breathing . . . on counting, on imagining your safe place once again. . . . Allow your vision to come alive as you breathe. Remember and focus on all the images in your safe place. . . . Breathe in the peace and the safety. . . . Breathe out the fear.

Allow your senses to come alive again in this place. Remember how it looks. Remember all the detail . . . the color of the sky . . . the grass or trees or sand or water. . . . Remember your place of safety and how very beautiful it is. . . . As you continue breathing in safety and breathing out fear, remember the sounds of your safe place. . . . Remember how wonderful it smells. . . . Remember the sights—glance around at your house or structure of safe shelter, and see your waterfall or pool of healing water. . . . And over there, see your garden. . . . And remember . . . remember the beauty and the peace and the safety. . . . Sit as long as you need to, breathing in safety and peace, breathing out fear, as long as you need to. . . . Do whatever else you need to do in your place of safety. Spend as long as you like. . . . And when you are ready, simply count yourself out by counting from one to five. And as you leave the place of safety, bring with you the knowing that you are safe . . . you are at peace . . . and everything is going to be all right.

IMAGERY FOR REDUCING PAIN

Allow yourself to be in a comfortable position, either lying down or sitting up. Make sure that your body is comfortable and well supported. Begin to take a couple of long, deep, cleansing breaths all the way down into your diaphragm. (Inhale.) Hold it, and as you exhale, let go of the tension. (Exhale.) Letting go. . . . Take another deep breath all the way in. (Inhale.) Allow all the tension to move into your lungs and then let it go (exhale), just begin to let go. . . . And if you're still feeling tense, repeat that process a few times as you begin to let go, begin to relax. . . . Create a silent and healing space around you. . . . Focus only on your quiet breathing and the sound of my voice. . . . Allow yourself to begin to let go, to create a healing time, a time to let go of pain.

As you lie there or sit quietly, imagine the light that fills you . . . fills your body from the crown of your head to the tips of your toes and fingers. . . . You can sense exactly where your pain is located in the vastness of your light. . . . Sensing it there for now, begin to draw this light up from your toes, as though leaving behind the dark . . . drawing the light up, condensing it as it moves up through your ankles and calves. . . . Draw it up through your knees and thighs. . . . As it condenses, pull the light up from your thighs through your pelvic area and hips . . . drawing it up and condensing the light into your belly. . . . Sense it there. All of the light from your legs and hips up in your belly. . . . Sense it there. . . . Now, begin to pull the light down from the crown of your head. . . . Sense it pulling down through the middle of your head and down your face . . . down to your chin, pulling down from your ears to the upper part of your neck and throat . . . condensing the light, sensing it moving down your neck and throat . . . pulling it down to your shoulders . . . condensing it there. . . . Now pull the light up from your fingertips to the palms of your hands . . . to your wrists. . . . Pulling the light up through your wrists and forearms all the way to your elbows . . . drawing it up and condensing it up to your upper arms, and finally joining the other light in your shoulders. . . . Now pull and condense all the light from your shoulders and upper chest. . . . Drawing it down, condensing it, pulling the light down to the light in your belly . . . where you condense it to a smaller and smaller ball of light in your belly . . . smaller and smaller to a ball of light, all of your light, all of your essence. . . .

Now send that ball of light to the place in your body where

you are experiencing pain right now. . . . Allow the ball of light to expand or contract to be the right size to surround and illuminate the pain. . . . See the pain, see what color it is . . . what shape and size it is. . . . See it surrounded in your light. . . . Now, mobilize the ball of light with the pain inside. . . . Begin to move it slowly so you can release it from your body. You may begin to move it toward an arm or leg to release from a hand or foot; you may move it toward the skin above the area. . . . Slowly move the ball of light with the pain inside . . . sense it moving . . . feeling it move . . . even feeling the pain in the new place. . . . Feeling the pain surrounded in a ball of light, moving slowly toward a hand or foot or up to the skin. . . . Slowly sense the ball of light beginning to emerge from your body . . . now gently resting on the surface of your skin. . . . When you are ready, shake it away or allow it to simply float away . . . you can sense it floating up through the room, up through the roof and out over the trees out of sight.

Now sense a tiny beam of new light, touching the crown of your head. You can feel this tiny beam of light . . . with a slight pressure touching the crown of your head. . . . Allow this new light to penetrate the top of your head. . . . Sense a warm light flooding your head and face, down your neck and throat, down through your shoulders and chest, flooding light down your arms to your hands, down your belly, where the light divides and floods down your thighs, knees, calves, ankles, and feet. Feel the new light filling the area where you had pain . . . soothing it. . . . Leave the light filling your body. . . . Feel the calm and the peace. . . . Know that each and every time you practice this, you will have more and more success . . . more and more relief from discomfort. . . . Scan your body now for changes, and rest.

Stay in this place as long as you would like. . . . You may

drift off to sleep, or when you are ready, simply count yourself out by counting from one to five. When you reach the number five, your eyes will open. And you will be awake and alert and feeling better.

IMAGERY FOR SENSING THE LIGHT

(To the caregiver: This imagery is for the practice of sensing the heaviness of the body and the lightness of the light body. It is very comforting. It in no way hastens the dying process but encourages the dying person to feel more comfortable with being so much more than her body.)

Allow yourself to be in a comfortable position, either lying down or sitting up. Make sure that your body is well supported. Begin to take a couple of long, deep, cleansing breaths all the way down into your diaphragm. (Inhale.) Hold it, and as you exhale, let go of the tension. (Exhale.) Letting go. . . . Take another deep breath all the way in. (Inhale.) Allow all the tension to move into your lungs and then let it go (exhale), just begin to let go. . . . And if you're still feeling tense, repeat that process a few times as you begin to let go, begin to relax. . . . Create a silent and healing space around you. . . . Focus only on your quiet breathing and the sound of my voice. . . . Allow yourself to begin to let go, to create a healing time, a time to explore the light. . . .

As you are lying there, sense the position of your body on the bed. . . . Feel where your skin touches the bottom sheet . . . all the places the sheet touches your skin. . . . Sense your body going deeper into the sheet and feel the fullness of the mattress under the sheet. . . . As you lie there comfortably, feel your body relaxing more and more and feeling supported by the bed. . . .

Off in the corner of your eye, sense a small ball of light . . . a small ball of light just to the side of you. . . . As the tiny ball of light moves just in front of you, sense it there. . . . Sense the tiny ball of light glowing and becoming larger . . . right in front of your eyes. . . . A beautiful ball of light that is so inviting, you want to touch it and feel its love. . . . Sensing the love in this ball of light, you feel a warmth of love welling up in your heart. . . . Feel the love in your heart. . . . Sense the love in the ball of light that is so inviting. . . . Feel the love in your heart that swells and forms its own light. . . . Send a beam of light from your heart to touch this ball of light . . . and the connection is good. . . . You can sense the flow of love back and forth from the light to your heart . . . and it feels so very good. . . .

Keeping this beam of light in place, feel a beam of light extending from your belly to the light . . . and the connection is good. . . . Feel the flow of light back to your belly from the light. . . . And with it comes safety and peace. . . . You can sense the flow of safety and peace back and forth from the light to your belly. . . . And with it you feel safety and peace . . . and it feels so very good. . . .

Keeping both beams of light in place . . . feel a beam of light from the crown of your head to the ball of light . . . and the connection is good. . . . Feel the flow of light back to the crown of your head from the light. . . . And with it comes a spiritual presence more beautiful than you have ever felt . . . more beautiful . . . and more real. . . . You can sense the flow of spirit back and forth from the light to the crown of your head. . . . Feel the beauty and the love of Spirit . . . and it feels so very good. . . .

Sense your body growing heavier and the real you growing lighter. . . . As your body becomes heavier . . . your light body becomes lighter. . . . You feel your light body becoming lighter. . . . You find yourself lifting . . . slowly lifting . . . lifting yourself toward the ball of light . . . following the three beams of light . . . bringing with you safety . . . love . . . and your spirit. . . . Feel yourself lifting into the light . . . experience! . . . the love . . . the peace. . . .

Stay in this place as long as you would like. . . . Whenever you like, you may leave the light and return to your resting body. . . . And return to the light whenever you are ready.

Suggested Spiritual Reading ∞

Anderson, Sherry Ruth, and Patricia Hopkins. *The Feminine Face of God.* Bantam Books, 1991.

Borysenko, Joan. *Fire in the Soul.* Warner Books, 1992.

Fowler, George. *Dance of a Fallen Monk.* Addison-Wesley Publishing Co., 1995.

Frankl, Victor E. *Man's Search for Meaning.* Pocket Books, 1959.

Fremantle, Francesca, and Chögyam Trungpa. *The Tibetan Book of the Dead.* Shambhala Publications, 1975.

Green, Arthur. *Seek My Face, Speak My Name.* Jason Aronson, 1992.

Harrison, Gavin. *In the Lap of the Buddha.* Shambhala Publications, 1994.

Henricks, Robert, trans., and Lao-Tzu. *Te-Tao Ching.* Ballantine Books, 1989.

Kapleau, Philip. *The Wheel of Life and Death.* Anchor Books, 1989.

Kushner, Harold S. *When Bad Things Happen to Good People.* Avon Books, 1981.

Kushner, Lawrence. *God Was in This Place, and I, i Did Not Know.* Jewish Lights Publishing, 1991.

Lewis, C. S. *A Grief Observed.* Bantam Books, 1963/1976.

McNeill, John J. *Freedom, Glorious Freedom.* Beacon Press, 1995.

Mitchell, Stephen. *The Book of Job.* North Point Press, 1979.

Monette, Paul. *Love Alone.* St. Martin's Press, 1988.

———. *West of Yesterday, East of Summer.* St. Martin's Press, 1994.

Moore, Thomas. *Care of the Soul.* HarperCollins, 1992.

Sogyal, Rinpoche. *Glimpse After Glimpse.* HarperSanFrancisco, 1995.

———. *The Tibetan Book of Living and Dying.* HarperSanFrancisco, 1992.

Sonsino, Rifat, and Daniel B. Syme. *What Happens After I Die?* UAHC Press, 1990.

Thompson, Mark. *Gay Soul.* HarperSanFrancisco, 1994.

Weems, Ann. *Psalms of Lament.* Westminster John Knox Press, 1995.

Wolpe, David J. *The Healer of Shattered Hearts.* Penguin Books, 1990.

Zukav, Gary. *The Seat of the Soul.* Simon & Schuster, 1990.

Selected Readings on Dying and Bereavement ✿

Aldrich, Sandra. *Living Through the Loss of Someone You Love.* Regal Books, 1990.

Ansley, Helen Green. *Life's Finishing School.* Institute of Noetic Sciences, 1990.

Berman, Claire. *Caring for Yourself While Caring for Your Aging Parents.* Henry Holt & Co., 1996.

Buckman, Robert. *I Don't Know What to Say.* Vintage Books, 1988.

Buscaglia, Leo. *The Fall of Freddie the Leaf.* Henry Holt & Co., 1982.

Colgrove, Melba, Harold H. Bloomfield, and Peter McWilliams. *How to Survive the Loss of a Love.* Bantam Books, 1976.

Doty, Mark. *Heaven's Coast.* HarperCollins, 1996.

Eadie, Betty J. *Embraced by the Light.* Bantam Books, 1992.

Fitzgerald, Helen. *The Mourning Handbook.* Fireside Books, 1994.

Froman, Paul Kent. *After You Say Goodbye.* Chronicle Books, 1992.

Jamison, Stephen. *Final Acts of Love.* Jeremy P. Tarcher, 1995.

Kramer, Kay and Herbert. *Conversations at Midnight.* Avon Books, 1993.

Kübler-Ross, Elisabeth. *Death Is of Vital Importance.* Station Hill Press, 1995.

———. *Death: The Final Stage of Growth.* Prentice-Hall, 1975.

———. *Living with Death and Dying.* Macmillan, 1981.

———. *On Children and Death.* Macmillan, 1983.

———. *On Death and Dying.* Macmillan, 1969.

———. *Questions and Answers on Death and Dying.* Macmillan, 1974.

Levine, Stephen. *Healing into Life and Death.* Anchor Books, 1987.

———. *Meetings at the Edge.* Anchor Books, 1984.

Lord, Janice. *Beyond Sympathy: What to Say and Do for Someone Suffering an Injury, Illness or Loss.* Pathfinder Publishers, 1988.

Moody, Raymond A. *Life After Life.* Bantam Books, 1975.

Munday, John, with Frances Wohlenhaus-Munday. *Surviving the Death of a Child.* Westminster John Knox Press, 1995.

Nuland, Sherwin. *How We Die.* Vintage Books, 1994.

Ritchie, Jean. *Death's Door.* Dell Publishing, 1994.

Sogyal, Rinpoche. *The Tibetan Book of Living and Dying.* HarperSanFrancisco, 1992.

Stasey, Bobbie. *Just Hold Me While I Cry: A Mother's Life-Enriching Reflections on Her Family's Emotional Journey Through AIDS.* Elysian Hills, 1993.

Temes, Roberta. *Living with an Empty Chair: A Guide Through Grief.* New Horizon Press, 1992.

Wakefield, Dan. *The Story of Your Life: Writing a Spiritual Autobiography.* Beacon Press, 1990.

Weenolsen, Patricia. *The Art of Dying.* St. Martin's Press, 1996.

Music for Healing

Adorjan, Andras, and Ayako Shinozaki. *Lyrical Melodies of Japan.* Nippon Columbia Co., 1992. DC 8114.

Aeoliah, *Angel Love.* Willow Tree. CD 033.

Boone, Steven. *Lazaris Remembers Lemuria.* NPN Publishing. (800) 678-2356.

———. *Through the Vortex.* NPN Publishing.

Crutcher, Rusty. *Machu Picchu Impressions.* Emerald Green Sound Productions, 1989. ED 8401.

Enya. *The Memory of Trees.* Reprise Records, a Time-Warner Company, 1995. 9-46106-2.

Erlien, Rick. *The Music of Yosemite.* Real Music, 1994. RM 1414.

Gibson, Dan. *Solitudes, Exploring Nature with Music: The Classics.* Dan Gibson Productions, 1991. CDG 104.

Goldmund, Boris. *Eklektik.* Boris Goldmund, 1989. 8-80001-2.

Goodall, Medwyn. *Earth Healer.* New World Music. NWCD 218.

———. *Merlin.* New World Co., 1990. NWCD 196.

———. *The Way of the Dolphin.* New World Music. NWC 220.

Gregorian Choir of Paris. *Gregorian Chant, Liturgy for Good Friday.* Licensed from Erato Editions, Costallat, 1985. MHS 11206.

Kater, Peter, and Carlos Nakai. *Migration.* Silver Wave Records. SD 704.

Kirkby, Emma, and Christopher Page. *A Feather on the Breath of God.* Hyperion Records, 1986. CDA 66039.

Korb, Ron, and Hiroki Sakaguchi. *Japanese Mysteries.* Oasis Productions, 1993. OASCD 1008.

Miles, Anthony. *Even Wolves Dream.* New World Co. NWDC 251.

Mock, Andreas. *Merlin's Magic.* Inner Worlds Music. CD 41025.

On Wings of Song and Robert Gass. *Heart of Perfect Wisdom/A Sufi Song of Love.* Spring Hill Music, 1993. SHM 6004.

Robertson, Kim. *Moonrise.* Invincible Music, 1987. INV 078.

Serrie, John. *And the Stars Go with You.* Miramar Recordings, 1987. MPCD 2.

Slap, Robert. *Atlantis: Crystal Chamber.* Inner Harmony New Age Music. CD 101.

———. *Atlantis: Healing Temple.* Inner Harmony New Age Music. CD 109.

Souther, Richard. *Vision, the Music of Hildegard von Bingen.* Angel Records, 1994. CDC 7243-5-55246-21.

Stagg, Hilary. *Beyond the Horizon.* Real Music, 1988. RM 1795.

———. *Dream Spiral.* Real Music, 1991. RM 1805.

———. *The Edge of Forever.* Real Music, 1993. RM 1810.

Any selection of nature sounds: oceans, streams, wind.

REFLEXOLOGY CHART

RIGHT FOOT **LEFT FOOT**

Brain
Sinus
Brain
Sinus
Brain
Sinus
Brain
Sinus
Brain
Sinus
Brain
Sinus
Sinus
Pituitary
Thyroid, Throat, Neck
Cervical spine
Eyes, Ears, Nose, Throat
Headache/Migraine and Sinus
Chest, Lymphatics, Lungs, Shoulders/Shoulder blades
Shoulders/Elbows
Solar plexus, Heart, Diaphragm
Thoracic spine
Liver
Gall bladder
Adrenal
Kidney
Pancreas
Transverse colon
Hip, Knee, Thigh
Appendix
Ileocecal valve
Ascending colon
Small intestines
Bladder
Lumbar spine
Reproductive
Reproductive
Lymphatics
Sciatica
Hip, Knee, Thigh
Sacrum
Coccyx

Brain
Sinus
Brain
Sinus
Brain
Sinus
Brain
Sinus
Brain
Sinus
Sinus
Thyroid, Throat, Neck
Eyes, Ears, Nose, Throat
Shoulders/Elbows
Solar plexus, Heart, Diaphragm
Stomach
Spleen
Adrenal
Kidney
Pancreas
Transverse colon
Hip, Knee, Thigh
Descending colon
Small intestines
Bladder
Sigmold colon
Rectum
Reproductive
Reproductive
Lymphatics
Sciatica
Hip, Knee, Thigh

Reflex points are the same for the top and bottom views of each foot.

Courtesy of Jeanette L. Golter, A.R.C., Board Certified Reflexologist.

Formats for Obituaries

The purpose of the obituary is to notify the public of the passing of your loved one and to give honor to the deceased by relating some of his personal accomplishments in life. Many people also retain a copy of the obituary as a memento.

The newspaper or journal in which the obituary appears will have certain rules or guidelines as to what is acceptable. For instance, in some publications the cause of death is not included; in others only spouses or blood relatives may be listed among the survivors. It is best to inquire before composing the obituary, to avoid hurt feelings and disappointment. We strongly advise that the obituary be either typed or printed in large block letters and delivered either personally or by fax, to avoid mistakes in the final copy.

The following are some examples of obituaries that have actually been used. You may adapt their format to conform to your particular requirements.

LAST NAME, FIRST NAME—age 44, passed away peacefully at home following a long struggle with (cause of death) on (date of death). Graduate of —— University and University of —— College of Law. Practiced law in —— from 1978 until 1988. Was Executive Director of ——, 1990. Member of —— Synagogue. Survived by longtime companion (name); brothers (name) and (name), their families, and many wonderful friends. Family and friends will meet at 10:45 A.M. at New Jewish Cemetery for 11 A.M. graveside service Sunday, August 21, Rabbi (name) officiating. Friends will be received at the home following the service. Memorials may be made to (name of organization with address). Arrangements by (name of mortuary).

LAST NAME, FIRST NAME—age 41, of ——, died (date), at Fort Sanders Regional Medical Center. He was a former employee of (name of company) in ——. Survivors: parents (names); brother (name); numerous aunts and uncles. Memorial service 8 P.M. Monday, Rose Highland Chapel. Memorials may be made to (name of organization with address). The family will receive friends 7–8 P.M. Monday at Rose Mortuary.

LAST NAME, FIRST NAME—age 61, resident of (name of town), died Saturday, (date) at (place of death). Member of St. Paul's Lutheran Church. Formerly employed at (place of employment). Active member and participant with (favorite organization or charity). Survivors: brothers (names and residences); several loving nieces and nephews; many devoted friends.

Memorial service 4 P.M. St. Paul's Church (give address, with name of officiating clergy if any). In lieu of flowers memorials may be made to (name of organization with address). (Name of mortuary).

It is a good idea to compose the obituary before the death occurs, even though it may seem morbid. After the death, the caregivers and survivors will be fully occupied with their grief and will have little energy to be creative.

About the Authors

Joan Furman, M.S.N., R.N., H.N.C.

Joan Furman is a nurse practitioner who offers counseling, healing touch therapies, guided imagery, and other approaches to create a healthful mind/body relationship. She works with people who suffer from cancer, HIV, and other life-threatening conditions as they heal and as they and their loved ones prepare for death.

She has published extensively in nursing and medical journals, newspapers, and magazines. Joan has served on the boards of community-based agencies, such as Alive Hospice, and other organizations and foundations at the local, state, national, and international levels. She has coordinated several statewide advisory committees to the governor of Tennessee, including the AIDS Advisory Committee.

Joan has degrees in psychology and nursing, is board-certified in holistic nursing, and is a Reiki master therapist/teacher. She has attended about 1,100 deaths in her twenty-eight years as a nurse practitioner. She teaches community health nursing and studies in holistic nursing to graduate students at Vanderbilt University.

David McNabb is a writer and AIDS activist now living in Denver, Colorado. He has been a lawyer in both private practice and government service.

David received his B.S. in 1975 and his M.A. in 1976 from Ball State University in Muncie, Indiana, and completed his legal studies at the University of Tennessee in Knoxville in 1979.

In 1987 he was appointed by the governor of Tennessee to service on the state's AIDS Advisory Committee, at which time he began caring for people with AIDS who were facing death.

David has been recognized by local, state, and national organizations for his service to people with AIDS. AIDS Response Knoxville honored him with several service awards, and in 1994 he was given a National Caregiver Award by the Family AIDS Network, Inc. He was a frequent lecturer on AIDS in Knoxville's church and school groups as well as a regular speaker at the AIDS course at the University of Tennessee. He served as an instructor in the buddy program of AIDS Response Knoxville, helped to found another AIDS program at Knoxville's Child and Family Services, and worked for the establishment of the Hope Center at Ft. Sanders Regional Medical Center in Knoxville, an agency serving the needs of people with AIDS.

David writes for *LGNY,* a newspaper in New York, and *Quest* magazine in Denver.

OTHER BELL TOWER BOOKS

*Books that nourish the soul, illuminate the mind,
and speak directly to the heart*

Valeria Alfeyeva
PILGRIMAGE TO DZHVARI
A Woman's Journey of Spiritual Awakening
An unforgettable introduction to the riches of the Eastern Orthodox mystical tradition. A modern *Way of a Pilgrim.*
0-517-88389-9 Softcover

Madeline Bruser
THE ART OF PRACTICING
Making Music from the Heart
A classic work on how to practice music which combines meditative principles with information on body mechanics and medicine.
0-517-70822-2 Hardcover

Melody Ermachild Chavis
ALTARS IN THE STREET
A Neighborhood Fights to Survive
For those who seek to put spirituality to work where it really counts—on the street where we live.
0-517-70492-7 Hardcover

Tracy Cochran and Jeff Zaleski
TRANSFORMATIONS
Awakening to the Sacred in Ourselves
An exploration of enlightenment experiences and the ways in which they can transform our lives.
0-517-70150-2 Hardcover

David A. Cooper
ENTERING THE SACRED MOUNTAIN
Exploring the Mystical Practices of Judaism, Buddhism, and Sufism
An inspiring chronicle of one man's search for truth.
0-517-88464-X Softcover

David A. Cooper
SILENCE, SIMPLICITY, AND SOLITUDE
A Guide for Spiritual Retreat
Required reading for anyone contemplating a retreat.
0-517-88186-1 Softcover

Marc David
NOURISHING WISDOM
A Mind/Body Approach to Nutrition and Well-Being
A book that advocates awareness in eating.
0-517-88129-2 Softcover

Kat Duff
THE ALCHEMY OF ILLNESS
A luminous inquiry into the function and purpose of illness.
0-517-88097-9 Softcover

Noela N. Evans
*MEDITATIONS FOR THE PASSAGES AND
CELEBRATIONS OF LIFE*
A Book of Vigils
Articulating the often unspoken emotions experienced at such times as
birth, death, and marriage.
0-517-59341-6 Hardcover
0-517-88299-X Softcover

Bernard Glassman and Rick Fields
INSTRUCTIONS TO THE COOK
A Zen Master's Lessons in Living a Life That Matters
A distillation of Zen wisdom that can be used equally well as a man-
ual on business or spiritual practice, cooking or life.
0-517-88829-7 Softcover

Burghild Nina Holzer
A WALK BETWEEN HEAVEN AND EARTH
A Personal Journal on Writing and the Creative Process
How keeping a journal focuses and expands our awareness of ourselves and
everything that touches our lives.
0-517-88096-2 Softcover

Greg Johanson and Ron Kurtz
GRACE UNFOLDING
Psychotherapy in the Spirit of the Tao-te ching
The interaction of client and therapist illuminated through the gentle
power and wisdom of Lao Tsu's ancient classic.
0-517-88130-6 Softcover

Selected by Marcia and Jack Kelly
ONE HUNDRED GRACES
Mealtime Blessings
A collection of graces from many traditions, inscribed in calligraphy rem-
iniscent of the manuscripts of medieval Europe.
0-517-58567-7 Hardcover
0-609-80093-0 Softcover

Jack and Marcia Kelly
SANCTUARIES
A Guide to Lodgings in Monasteries, Abbeys, and Retreats of the United States
For those in search of renewal and a little peace; described by the *New
York Times* as "the *Michelin Guide* of the retreat set."
THE NORTHEAST 0-517-57727-5 Softcover
THE WEST COAST & SOUTHWEST 0-517-88007-5 Softcover
THE COMPLETE U.S. 0-517-88517-4 Softcover

Marcia M. Kelly
HEAVENLY FEASTS
Memorable Meals from Monasteries, Abbeys, and Retreats
Thirty-nine celestial menus from the more than 250 monasteries the
Kellys have visited on their travels.
0-517-88522-0 Softcover

Barbara Lachman
THE JOURNAL OF HILDEGARD OF BINGEN
A year in the life of the twelfth-century German saint—the diary she
never had the time to write herself.
0-517-59169-3 Hardcover
0-517-88390-2 Softcover

Katharine Le Mée
CHANT
The Origins, Form, Practice, and Healing Power of Gregorian Chant
The ways in which this ancient liturgy can nourish us and transform our
lives.
0-517-70037-9 Hardcover

Stephen Levine
A YEAR TO LIVE
How to Live This Year as If It Were Your Last
Using the consciousness of our mortality to enter into a new and vibrant
relationship with life.
0-517-70879-5 Hardcover

Gunilla Norris
BECOMING BREAD
Meditations on Loving and Transformation
A book linking the food of the spirit—love—with the food of the body—
bread.
0-517-59168-5 Hardcover

Gunilla Norris
BEING HOME
A Book of Meditations
An exquisite modern book of hours, a celebration of mindfulness in
everyday activities.
0-517-58159-0 Hardcover

Ram Dass and Mirabai Bush
COMPASSION IN ACTION
Setting Out on the Path of Service
Heartfelt encouragement and advice for those ready to commit time and energy to relieving suffering in the world.
0-517-88500-X Softcover

His Holiness Shantanand Saraswati
THE MAN WHO WANTED TO MEET GOD
Myths and Stories that Explain the Inexplicable
The teaching stories of one of India's greatest living saints.
0-517-88520-4 Softcover

Rabbi Rami M. Shapiro
MINYAN
Ten Principles for Living Life of Integrity
A tenfold path for those interested to know what Judaism has to offer the spiritually hungry.
0-609-80055-8 Softcover

Rabbi Rami M. Shapiro
WISDOM OF THE JEWISH SAGES
A Modern Reading of Pirke Avot
A third-century treasury of maxims on justice, integrity, and virtue— Judaism's principal ethical scripture.
0-517-79966-9 Hardcover

Joan Tollifson
BARE-BONES MEDITATION
Waking Up from the Story of My Life
An unvarnished, exhilarating account of one woman's struggle to make sense of her life.
0-517-88792-4 Softcover

Richard Whelan, Ed.

SELF-RELIANCE

The Wisdom of Ralph Waldo Emerson as Inspiration for Daily Living

A distillation of Emerson's spiritual writings for contemporary readers.

0-517-58512-X Softcover

Bell Tower books are for sale at your local bookstore or you may call Random House at 1-800-793-BOOK to order with a credit card.